What I really love is the practical advice that Emma gives us to do on our own based on her experience working with athletes of all kinds (drummers, golfers, tennis players, etc) and how she dispels a few of the common practices that we have relied on in the past with little results.

Jeff Pelizzaro, host of the **18STRONG** podcast

I'm so grateful for having found Emma when I did and enrolling on to her program. It quickly put my mind in a more positive space with the light at the end of the tunnel that I needed. After just a month on the course, I was mostly pain-free day to day, and after 3 months I gradually started getting back to the activities I love.

Will Holland, Motorcycle Racer

Emma teaches the numerous potential causes for pain, the most effective ways to prevent and treat it, the 4 phases of healing, why it is important to normalize tension in your body before strengthening it, why you should use heat instead of ice after a few days of having pain, and much more!

Mehrban Iranshad, host of the **Tennis Files** podcast

Emma's value proposition is that she helps people get their life back and enables them to rojoin the activities they enjoy. She truly has a ton of expertise.

PragmaticInstitute.com

I saw Emma on the Tennis Summit and did part of her full-week mini-course. I thought they were both very good.

Tom Nordstrom MD, Orthopedic Surgeon

Praise for *Tennis Elbow Relief*

Emma is definitely the QUEEN

A great guide that will help anyone who is suffering from Tennis Elbow to get back in the game and back in their lives pain free!

Eimear Zone, Author of *The Little Book of Good Enough*

The only program I've seen that works for Tennis Elbow!

I can tell you that her strategies are not only things you have not heard before but flat work. Tennis elbow is difficult to treat if not impossible. Emma will get you on the path to recovery if you are patient and willing to put in the effort.

Todd B. Bondy

Excellent resource for tennis elbow sufferers

This book contains all the information you need to heal your tennis elbow. It is an invaluable resource if you are suffering from tennis elbow symptoms. Cannot recommend highly enough to those wishing to get healed effectively and fully.

William Holland

The only thing that works!

I have attended many programs of tennis elbow online from other therapists and wasted thousands of dollars. I am thankful to God that I came across Emma Green and her book. The depth of knowledge she has on tennis elbow is unparalleled to any other physical therapist out there. Believe me, I have seen a lot of therapists. After using the strategies outlined in the book, I am already feeling much better and my symptoms have completely resolved. I am back to doing all my favorite activities. I wish I had found Emma earlier.

Ankit Gupta

I had been suffering pain in both elbows, one side was worse than the other. It was ongoing for months and even the smallest touch on my elbows was so incredibly painful. I followed very sensible and pragmatic advice from the book and can honestly say within a few weeks my pain has substantially improved.

Bronah B.

I am 54 years old, use a keyboard for a living and am an avid tennis player. 4 months ago, I was devastated to realize that I had an overuse injury that took me away from tennis completely. I had tennis elbow. As a result, I bought Emma's book and couldn't wait to read it. I am amazed at the difference following Emma's protocol has made. I am back on court doing footwork training and hitting lightweight balls. More importantly I am doing exercises off court to strengthen and improve more than just my elbow and I can now see steady improvements in my grip strength (gone from 40lbs to 80lbs) and strength in all my arm/ shoulders and core. Now I see the light at the end of the tunnel and I'm also more knowledgeable about how to manage / strengthen my body. I can't thank Emma enough. If you are struggling with elbow pain and grip / arm weakness. I strongly recommend this book.

Susie Q

Tired of suffering from Tennis Elbow & more? Best foundation for full healing without meds/surgery!
After 10 months of recurring pain and visits with many different specialists and tests! I was tired of the chronic pain and suffering, there has to be someone out there who can help. Wish I had this book and info from the start! This book is a foundation of expertise, experience, and genuine caring and healing. She explains the stages of repair and healing so that I can understand what I am feeling and going through and what to expect. Her program is phenomenal if you are looking to fully heal without meds or surgery, worth every penny for full recovery and no wasted time/appts. Brilliant PT!

Mommie P

Great resource for clinicians and patients

As a licensed physical therapist of 10+ years, I am always looking for additional resources to gain knowledge and add to my skill set. This was such a refreshing read that accounted for treating the entire body as a whole instead of just the isolated injury. You don't have to be a physical therapist or have a medical background to understand this book as it is written in a clear way that anyone can understand. Highly recommended to clinicians and patients.

Grateful for this resource

As someone who has suffered with tennis elbow for years, Emma lays out the exact solution to my problem. I have seen endless doctors, physical therapists and occupational therapists and no one has laid out this type of healing plan to me before.

The gratitude and love I feel for Emma is many levels deep. I'm thrilled that the techniques she created for my issues have helped so many people overcome their own elbow problems. It wasn't always easy, but it was miraculous for me. I'll always be indebted to, and thankful for, the tiny English woman who healed my elbow. My friend, "the Tennis Elbow Queen", Emma Green.

Buddy Gibbons, Drummer, Composer, Producer

Tennis Elbow Relief

Serving up solutions for lateral epicondylitis

Also, by Emma Green

Get Out of Pain FAST! –
Your Healing Guidebook

Tennis Elbow Relief 2.0: Serving up solutions for lateral epicondylitis
Author: Emma Green

Published by: Emma Green Programs

California, USA

www.tenniselbowqueen.com

The information provided in this book is designed to provide helpful information on the subjects discussed. This book is not meant to be used, nor should it be used, to diagnose or treat any medical condition. For diagnosis or treatment of any medical problem, consult your own physician.

ISBN (paperback):   978-1-7368460-3-2
ISBN (hardback):   978-1-7368460-4-9
ISBN (eBook):   978-1-7368460-5-6

Cover design & formatting and interior book design & formatting by Leesa Ellis of 3 ferns > www.3ferns.com

$1 from the sale of this book goes to support the amazing work of Dachshunds and Friends Rescue. "A home for every dog and a dog for every home."

Emma Green
The Tennis Elbow Queen

presents

Tennis Elbow Relief 2.0

Serving up solutions
for lateral epicondylitis

**Learn the fundamental steps
that take you from hurt to healed!**

Essential reading for people who are
ready to resolve elbow pain for good.

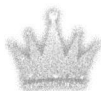

Emma Green
PROGRAMS

My boys – I am so proud of you.

My family, for supporting me through everything I want to achieve.

My clients, without whom, this book wouldn't exist.

"You are the reason I do what I do. You are the reason I work every day.

To see you recover from debilitating injuries, witnessing your transformations, and regaining the lives you want to live is a gift.

I am truly humbled to share this journey with you and honored that you entrust me with your care."

TENNIS ELBOW QUEEN

Contents

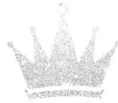

Welcome

Welcome to a growing group of people who are taking their health into their own hands and healing themselves. They may have tried many other solutions in the past, but nothing seemed to help. So, they took responsibility and searched out a better way to heal themselves.

Within the pages of this book, you will find many strategies to resolve lateral epicondylitis, also known as tennis elbow. Some of them you will most likely have tried before, and some will be new to you. Trust the process. This program has worked for thousands of people all over the world and is now in a format to help you. I wanted to write a book that someone could pick up and heal their tennis elbow themselves.

There are several bonuses in downloadable form. However, they are not mandatory. You'll still find all the information in the book. To get access to the extra resources I mention, sign up for free at:

https://bit.ly/TE-bookbonuses

Although we are not directly working together, I'm here with you on this journey. I've included links to my website and Facebook group to aid you in your journey to healing. But as I mentioned, these are not required. Just think of them as optional extras. Everything you need to heal is covered in this book alone. However, don't hesitate to reach out if you have any questions. I LOVE questions!

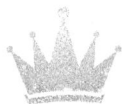

Preface to the Second Edition

WHAT'S NEW

Welcome to the second edition of *Tennis Elbow Relief: Serving Up Solutions For Lateral Epicondylitis.*

Why a second edition?

Firstly, because you asked for it! It became evident that all the strategies needed to be in the book. The first edition had several videos accompanying the book – if a picture tells a thousand words, then a video surely must tell ten thousand! I assumed it would be easier for readers to follow the exercises in video format, but evidently, that was not the case for everyone. I fully appreciate this as I have done the same thing as some of my readers; I get into bed at night and start reading a book. It directs me to a link for bonuses; a quiz, or something similar and I think I'll do that in the morning. The next evening, I get into bed and reach for the book. It's only when I open the pages, I realize that I didn't follow up on the link! D'oh! I think to myself, oh well, I'm not going to do it now, so I'll wait until the following day... This scenario repeats itself ad infinitum! I get you, reader! Hence a thicker book and not having to find videos through a different link if you don't want to.

This has also led to a revised structure of the book. The chapters have been rearranged slightly. You need to be able to find the most salient points and implement them ASAP. So, you'll find the most important points at the beginning of each chapter, followed by the research.

This allows you to skip through the book, gaining the information you need for healing, but then you can dive deeper into the research if you are wondering why you are doing a particular strategy.

Talking of research, the original research articles from the first edition are included by number. However, additional references new to the second edition are cited and alphabetized in the references section at the back of the book for clarity on what's been added.

Additionally, medical research has changed rapidly in some areas, and new elements have been added to the program. These are incredibly helpful in calming the nervous system and are essential for the fastest possible healing of a tendon issue like tennis elbow.

In summary, I've simplified the formula to make it easier to follow and implement. But don't worry, I'm still here to answer your questions should any arise, just reach out to:

Emma@TennisElbowQueen.com

So, without further ado, let's hear from someone who was instrumental in the formation of this program. But for them, this book wouldn't be in your hands right now!

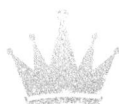

Foreword

BY BUDDY GIBBONS

am a professional drummer. You've heard me play on thousands of television commercials, broadcasts, sports shows, and film scores. You've never heard OF me, but you've heard me.

But that almost wasn't my life at all.

The year was 2008. My wife and I had moved to Los Angeles after a stint in Nashville. I knew that I had to work incredibly hard to establish myself in the uber-competitive LA music scene. I searched out work in every nook and cranny of the Craigslist, the *LA Weekly*, *The Recycler*, and I took every gig that I could... over 300 of them. I began having some trouble with my right arm... numbness, tingling, pain. Eventually, the pain became so intense that I could no longer lift a bottle of water. I had to hug a pillow any time I was sitting, just so that I could keep my arm in a specific position where it didn't hurt quite as badly. As you can imagine, that made things quite difficult for someone in my line of work. I had played my arm to death. It was time to seek medical help.

I began with my general practitioner. She couldn't figure out what the problem was because my symptoms didn't perfectly match any of the syndromes/problems/injuries she was familiar with. So, we decided to go the route of cortisone shots. Over the next year and a half, I had so many shots that I actually considered getting an "X" tattooed on the spot where my elbow pain originated. I figured I could take out the guesswork that way. But the reality was that the shots weren't a cure, they were only a treatment, and my career was in serious jeopardy. I sought out a surgeon and ran across some seriously questionable ideas about fixing my elbow, not the least of which was the suggestion by a doctor who wanted to take a hammer and chisel to my bones, only to give me a 70% chance of recovery. No thanks! Finally, I met a truly caring surgeon in Pasadena, and she said to me, "I can't fix your elbow, but I have an idea..." That idea was to get me into Occupational Therapy.

My Occupational Therapist was a wonderful person, and I could tell that she was both sympathetic and empathetic to my situation. We worked for several months, with little to no change in my pain level and functionality. My body had begun to shut down in other ways as well. Muscles were tightening all over my body. I was no longer moving in a normal manner at all. Photos taken of me during that time show that I was wearing 'pain face' everywhere I went. I still have a hard time looking at pictures from that time in my life. In the meantime, my case became something of a talking point in the hospital's therapy department. It was finally determined that the best chance I had for recovery was to move from occupational therapy to physical therapy.

Enter, Emma Green.

Long before she was 'The Tennis Elbow Queen', she was just the latest person in whom I was putting my hope. My previous experience with Physical Therapy had not been particularly positive, but I was desperate for help. She walked into the room, this tiny English lady, with a charming smile and a deeply caring demeanor. I could feel how much interest she had in me and my case. Beyond her obvious 'care', however, was a keenly curious mind. She wanted to figure me out. She wanted to help me.

We began my therapy sessions... they did not go well. I was getting quite frustrated because, for the first few weeks, we never touched my elbow. Finally, in my despair, I asked her to PLEASE explain to me why we were working on my back... my shoulder... my big toe (not really)! So, she calmly took me down the hall to meet "Henry", the life-sized, half-muscle, half-bone skeleton in the other exam room. She showed me how my muscles, tendons, ligaments, and bones connected to each other, and how one movement was part of the bigger picture of many movements. My neck and back were so tight that there was no way my elbow would be able to heal until she got the rest of my body moving the correct way. From that moment on, I knew that, no matter how long it took, I was going to be ok. She really did understand. She saw the big picture.

A few weeks went by and I achieved a modicum of progress on my neck and shoulders. In fact, I could now turn my head like a normal person! Then it happened: "Buddy, I've got an idea". I was certain I'd heard that line before. So what, exactly, was Emma's idea? She had devised a therapy for the elbow based on the science of repairing an Achilles tendon. She explained in great detail how she could see the principles of the Achilles treatment working to repair the damage inside my elbow.

So, we began. Day one, she showed me the exercise. I was skeptical. After all, what good would an exercise with a 1lb weight do for me, a 6'2", 230lb, athletically built man? I scoffed at the idea... until I couldn't complete the movement with that small amount of weight. That's how damaged my elbow was. That's how much pain I was in. She instructed me to go home and do that exercise twice a day, three sets. It was difficult to admit just how weak I was. It was embarrassing. It was frustrating, but I did the work. Eventually, I could get through the sets with one pound. Then two pounds. I began to feel a little bit of relief. I didn't hurt constantly. I didn't have to sleep with a pillow tucked into my arm every single night. Each visit with Emma, she'd measure my grip strength and put me through the paces of the exercise. She'd still mobilize my back and shoulders, she'd push me to increase the weight.

Then came 'that' Tuesday morning. I'll never forget it. I'd gotten up and was fixing myself a bowl of Cap'n Crunch. I reached into the refrigerator, took out the milk, poured it over the cereal, replaced the milk in the fridge, and closed the door… with my damaged right arm! I had no pain at all. In fact, it felt so natural that I didn't realize what I'd done until I was halfway into the living room with my prized sugary treat! When it hit me, I sat the bowl down, again with my right arm, and began to sob. I called my wife and told her what had happened. She cried at her office. We celebrated that night as if it was the biggest news we'd ever gotten. Why?

Because that was the moment I got my life back.

It's been over a decade now, and my elbow is still as good as new. If I ever feel any issues coming on, I turn to the exercises Emma created for me and I'm back to 100% within a day or two. The gratitude and love I feel for Emma is many levels deep. I'm thrilled that the techniques she created for my issues have helped so many other people overcome their own elbow problems. It wasn't always easy, but it was miraculous for me.

I'll always be indebted to, and thankful for, the tiny English woman who healed my elbow. My friend, "The Tennis Elbow Queen", Emma Green.

– **Buddy Gibbons**

Drummer • Composer • Producer

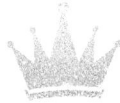

Introduction

Hello. I'm Emma Green, the Tennis Elbow Queen! I'm actually a physical therapist, or physiotherapist as we are known in some parts of the world. I was born, raised, and trained in the UK, working there for a little over 11 years before relocating to the USA and getting my physical therapy license in California.

In the UK, I worked with several sports teams and traveled globally, helping athletes compete at the very highest level. When I moved to the USA and had two kids, the traveling slowed. My practice also changed from working with professional athletes to working with professional musicians. They didn't need me to travel with them, but their mindset, drive, and work ethic were no different from the athletes I was so used to helping. What was different, though, was the type of injuries I was seeing. The athletes I worked with would injure their backs, knees, and ankles, while the musicians would complain about their necks, shoulders, and elbows.

After an incredibly comprehensive education at a large regional teaching hospital in the National Health Service in the UK, I spent 6 months working alongside a Shoulder Consultant and a further 6 months in a specialist hand unit. This gave me great insight into musicians' movement patterns and mechanisms of injury.

This new direction began when I was asked by a coworker, who is a Certified Hand Therapist, to assess a professional drummer she was treating for tennis elbow. The drummer, Buddy (he tells his story in the foreword to this book), was desperate for answers to his problem as he couldn't play and so couldn't make a living and anyone who knows a musician knows that making music is not just what they do, but it's who they are. Buddy had had that taken away from him.

He was truly miserable and borderline depressed. He and his wife had traveled the country looking for a solution to his tennis elbow and had failed. Acupuncture, chiropractic treatment, massage, stretches, doctors, cortisone shots... nothing worked. He ended up in a surgeon's office begging for surgery to alleviate his pain. Thankfully, she refused until he had seen one of her trusted therapists, that is, the Certified Hand Therapist I shared an office with at the time.

After I evaluated Buddy, it became patently clear that there was way more going on than "just a tennis elbow." How many times have you heard that phrase from people who have clearly never suffered from tennis elbow?

During the time I worked with Buddy, I trawled the research to come up with the very best, latest, and most evidence-based treatments for tendon healing that I could find. There was nothing there for tennis elbow. The research was very good at telling us what didn't work, but not as good at telling us what did. So, I used my sports background knowledge to devise a brand-new program, something that had never been seen before, to treat Buddy and get him back to doing what he loves, playing the drums.

After he healed, he happily went back to the surgeon's office for a check-up appointment. She called me soon after and asked me what new treatments I was doing that had been so effective for someone who had been told there was a strong chance he would never likely be able to play the drums again. I shared with her my program and a strong working relationship was born. She still sends me her tennis elbow patients to this day over 15 years after I first worked with Buddy. I'm proud to call her a friend.

Who is this book for?

This book is for anyone who is suffering from tennis elbow. Anyone feeling pain on the outside of their elbow and/or down their forearm. Research shows that up to 3% of the adult population will suffer from tennis elbow at some point in their lives.[1]

My first recollection of the term "tennis elbow" came as a child. My Mum was diagnosed with lateral epicondylitis (tennis elbow) probably due to looking after 3 kids and keeping house, and the treatment she was given was a cortisone injection, nothing else, no therapy, no exercises, just straight in with a shot. I can remember her saying it was the most painful thing she had ever endured, and she'd had 3 children. Sadly, her pain came back, and she underwent another injection. Boy, tennis elbow must be pretty bad if someone went through 2 intensely painful injections to try to resolve it.

I guess that's why I subconsciously did everything in my power to help Buddy heal. When I met him, I was in a position to utilize my skills to solve his problem, something that my Mum had been unable to find years before. That's how my Tennis Elbow Relief program came into being. It's been refined over the years as new research has come out, and it's evolved to be effective as a remote treatment option having helped sufferers all over the world.

This book is for anyone who has searched for a solution to their tennis elbow pain but has failed. There's a ton of information out there regarding this subject and, unfortunately, not all of it is correct. Here I take you through the whats, whys, and wherefores of working towards resolving your own tennis elbow.

But first, what's in a name?

Tennis elbow is the layman's term for the problem that you have with your elbow. The most common medical terminology for tennis elbow is lateral epicondylitis. It can also be described as lateral epicondylosis, lateral epicondylopathy, or even lateral elbow pain. These all essentially mean the same thing. So, throughout this book, I will generally refer to this pathology as tennis elbow, its most commonly used name. Unless a specific research paper has used a particular terminology, in which case, I will use the terminology they chose. (As a side note, there are several direct quotes from research papers. As such you may notice a mixture of British and American spelling.)

If you have golfer's elbow, medial epicondylitis, medial epicondylosis, medial epicondylopathy, or medial elbow pain, many of the principles I describe in this book will help you, too. There are just a couple of subtle differences in the stretch and strengthening exercise used to treat it specifically. The same is true for biceps or triceps tendon problems. Follow the principles in this book, and don't hesitate to reach out if you have specific questions about your particular issue.

Let's get started...

TENNIS ELBOW
QUEEN

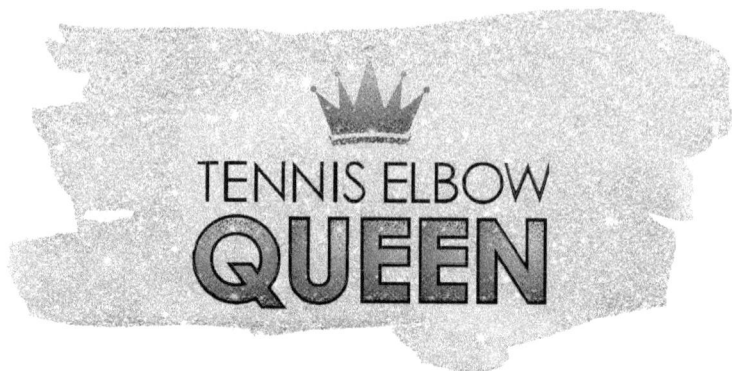

"After just a week my elbow is not hurting sharply like it was. I love the stretches and am now able to sleep comfortably through the night."

LR 34

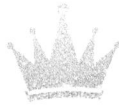

CHAPTER 1

Could Everything You've Been Told About Tennis Elbow Be Wrong?

The short answer would be... yes. However, to explain a little further and start to understand why some of these legends have evolved, I've picked out a few of the most commonly heard myths surrounding tennis elbow.

There's a lot of misinformation out there regarding lateral epicondylitis or tennis elbow and I guess it's because so many of us have either suffered from it at some point or another or know someone who has. The US Department of Health and Human Services, National Institutes of Health, cite that 1–3% of people will suffer from Tennis Elbow pain at some point in their lives.[2] The average general physical therapist, who sees everything and everybody, backs, necks, knees, elbows, and so on, generally sees one or two tennis elbow patients per year, So, that statistic is likely accurate. My team's caseload is a little different with over 80% of our clients suffering from tennis elbow.

How best to treat it? Just Google "tennis elbow treatment" if you haven't already and count the list of suggestions you get. It's infinite. How do you know what's right for you? Great question. How do you know if something's wrong for you? Even better question. You browse for a few minutes and then what? You do nothing. It's ok, we all do it. It's called Analysis Paralysis; too many options cause you to become overwhelmed, so you don't do any of them. Best to keep yourself safe, right? You think, "I'll just see how it goes..." Wait... what? Do you think it's going to suddenly and miraculously get better, even though you've been suffering with it for weeks, months, or even years?

Once you start telling people you've got tennis elbow or you put a strap on your arm and people see you've got tennis elbow, they're going to give you advice; all the things they've heard, the old wives' tales, the myths. Here are the top myths that clients have told me over the years.

1. It can't be tennis elbow – I don't play tennis
2. All tennis players get tennis elbow
3. Rest it and it will go away by itself eventually
4. A steroid injection will cure it
5. If injections don't work, surgery is the only option
6. You've got it for life, there's nothing you can do, you'll just have to live with it and take pain pills.
7. You only get it in your dominant arm...but then it will spread to the other arm
8. Anti-inflammatory medication helps as the elbow has been inflamed for months
9. It's your age
10. Your parents had it, so it'll be the same for you
11. You need an X-ray or an MRI scan to see what's wrong

12. Exercise will make it worse and you're in too much pain to come to therapy
13. Physical therapy (physiotherapy) doesn't work for tennis elbow
14. Virtual treatment won't work for tennis elbow

Do any of these sound familiar? Let's take a deeper look at them in turn.

1. It can't be tennis elbow – I don't play tennis

Mythbuster: Cutts et al (2019) stated *"tennis elbow is also seen in laborers who utilize heavy tools or engage in repetitive gripping or lifting tasks."*

Between 1–3% of the general population will suffer from tennis elbow at some point in their lives.[2]

This is the number one thing people say regarding tennis elbow. "How can I have tennis elbow? I don't play tennis!" In fact, most people who are suffering from tennis elbow, have never picked up a racket in their lives. The large majority of people suffering from tennis elbow develop it over time, from overuse of other activities, such as painting their house, using a screwdriver, playing a musical instrument, traveling, repetitive lifting at work or at home, housework, cleaning, renovating a property, increasing or changing their workout in the gym, repetitive movements at work, excessive computer use, keyboarding or mouse use, prolonged tablet or phone use...the list goes on and on.

2. All tennis players get tennis elbow

Mythbuster: Cutts et al (2019) stated *"up to 50% of all tennis players develop symptoms due to various factors including poor swing technique and the use of heavy racquets."*

But interestingly only 5% of professional tennis players will suffer, despite the high number of hours they play. This indicated that poor technique plays a large role in the 50% of non-professional players who develop elbow pain.

Have you ever played tennis? Or are you a tennis player? Of the thousands of tennis elbow sufferers, I've seen probably 40% are tennis players. Around 60% play some kind of racket sport, maybe not tennis, but racquetball, squash, badminton or pickleball.

A tennis coach once told me that he considers tennis elbow in tennis players to be "Bad Stroke-itis", meaning that people who use poor form while playing tennis are the ones who develop tennis elbow. This can be true, but it can also occur from simple overuse, even with a good technique. If someone jumped from playing tennis occasionally to suddenly playing for 8 hours every day, the tissues involved in gripping and swinging the racket would complain about how much extra work they were having to do, while not being used to it. You would ache like mad if you went and worked out hard at the gym if you weren't used to it. However, you do not have to play tennis to get tennis elbow. The good news is that no matter how you developed tennis elbow, the same program will resolve it.

3. Rest it and it will go away by itself, eventually

Mythbuster: Coombes et al (2013) found that *"the symptoms of lateral epicondylitis could persist for many years and relapses are very common."*

Rest from any aggravating activities is an important part of healing tennis elbow. However, rest itself will not cure tennis elbow and get the sufferer back doing all the activities they have been missing out on. The reason most people suffer from tennis elbow for such a long time is that the muscles involved become weak. Therefore, each time you use the muscle, more force goes through the injured tendon. Then, because it hurts, you do it less. If you do that activity less, the tendon doesn't get pulled on, but consequently, the attached muscle doesn't get used, leading to the muscle getting weaker and weaker the longer it's not used.

Continuing to stay away from any aggravating activity now gives the tendon a chance to start to resolve. Yay. You're heading in the right direction. But slow down, because once you feel a bit better, you might start to think about picking up the tennis racket, or whatever activity it happens to be that you are missing out on. You get excited at the prospect of getting back to normal and returning to all the fun things you love to do. But as soon as you try to lift the heavy saucepan, or whatever activity makes you happy, you feel that familiar pain, and your arm feels incredibly weak. Because it is. You've rested from irritating activities for long enough so that the tendon is no longer irritated, but because the muscles haven't been working out and they are still super weak, the structure cannot tolerate the stresses and strains of normal daily activities that you are now starting to do. So, guess what? The tendon starts to become irritated again... Vicious cycle . . .

Rest will help, absolutely it will. Relative rest is helpful for tennis elbow, but total rest is not going to cure it. It's a much better idea to keep moving and doing comfortable activities as your body tells you. Our bodies are very perceptive, we should listen to them more often.

Rest will decrease your symptoms. I've heard sufferers say, "If I don't play tennis, work out, play my musical instruments, play with my kids, pick my kids up, lift the groceries, pick up a bottle of water... If I don't do those things, I'm fine." That doesn't sound like living to me. That's no fun. You will use rest as a strategy to reduce irritation in your elbow, but it isn't going to cure the problem.

Tennis elbow does not heal itself. Tendons are notoriously stubborn to resolve. The reason is due to the pathology of the tendon; it cannot recover by just resting it. Your symptoms can settle down, but you won't be back doing everything you want to do because the tendon has not healed. The pain will always come back if you don't heal it correctly and often it will feel worse each time it recurs. You'll learn the exercise that does heal the tendon later in the book.

4. A steroid injection will cure it

Mythbuster: Hay et al (1999) showed *"no long-term benefit of steroid injection in tennis elbow."*

If research has shown us this for years, why is it STILL the first line of treatment offered to many patients?

Research has shown that multiple injections of steroid (cortisone) into a soft tissue, can weaken the structure of the soft tissue and cause it to fail, not only leading to a prolonged healing time but also poorer outcomes.[3] That's obviously not good. So, if someone says to you, "Cortisone injections are the best treatment for tennis elbow", not only is that not true, but they actually slow down healing and lead to the tendon not being able to heal as effectively as if it hadn't undergone the injection. If you've ever been prescribed oral steroids for an infection, you may have noticed your body feeling good. Your joints don't ache and your elbow's ok. Steroids can do that and cortisone is a steroid. But, read on.

Back in the fifties, sports doctors found that if they injected steroids into the joints and soft tissues of football players who were injured, they could get them on the field every week, week in and week out. However, a few years later, the football players started to fall apart. Quite literally. It is now known that if you have too many cortisone shots into one area of your body, in your lifetime, the steroid can degrade the soft tissues.[4] It starts to break them down. Some players experienced tendon ruptures. The muscle tissue was also breaking down and their ligaments would start to degrade. The sports doctors were not happy about this and they started looking into what was happening to the players. They realized that it was the cortisone.

Unverferth and Olix, (1973) stated *"The repeated use of local steroid injections in the treatment of tenosynovitis in the active athlete is to be abandoned, not only because it masks the symptoms of tenosynovitis, giving the patient a false sense of security, but also because local injection of steroid decreases the tensile strength of tendon and predisposes it to complete rupture."*

Fast forward to today and most doctors are decreasing the number of steroid shots they are performing for tendon pathologies such as tennis elbow. The realization has become apparent that shots for tennis elbow don't resolve the pathology, they may just mask the pain for a few weeks before the original symptoms return with a vengeance. Add to this the possibility of side effects that may come with an invasive procedure like an injection, and it becomes clear why the administering of steroid injections for tennis elbow is not the optimum course of action.

It's a band-aid, not a cure, and there are possible side effects[5,6] such as;

- It can degrade the soft tissues including cartilage, tendon, and skin, and potentially cause tendon ruptures
- It's an invasive procedure, so it is possible to get an infection in the area
- Discoloration or depigmentation of the skin around the area can occur
- Fat atrophy – the steroid affects and reduces the subcutaneous fat just under the skin from the surrounding area and makes the little bump on the elbow look much more prominent
- Steroid flare, a temporary increase in pain at the injured site
- Temporary facial flushing
- Disturbed menstrual pattern
- Skin rash, including cellulitis
- Temporary blood sugar spike
- Thinning or death of nearby bone (osteoporosis or osteomyelitis)
- Nerve damage
- Increased risk of injury recurrence

As you can see, for many reasons, cortisone shots are not the best treatment for tennis elbow. Consequently, I am very conservative when it comes to invasive procedures such as these. I believe that you should have no more than three cortisone injections into any one part of your body in your entire lifetime – and that doesn't include tendons. The good thing is that to successfully heal tennis elbow you don't need steroid injections at all. This is an outdated form of treatment. There are far more effective non-invasive treatments that can completely resolve tennis elbow so that it doesn't return. I call that a win Win WIN. In case you are wondering about other types of injections; you'll learn about these in more detail in chapter 4.

5. Surgery is the only option

Mythbuster: Bateman et al (2019) showed that *"surgical interventions for tennis elbow are no more effective than nonsurgical or sham interventions."*

Surgery of any kind should always be the absolute last resort. The reason is that once a tissue has been cut, it will never be 100% again. Soft tissues that are cut repair themselves with scar tissue, not the original tissue. That is, muscle tissue doesn't heal with muscle tissue, it heals with scar tissue. Ligaments don't heal with ligament tissue; they heal with scar tissue. Cut tendons don't heal with tendon tissue, they heal with scar tissue.

This is important to understand because once a tissue heals with scar tissue it is not completely normal as there's an area of essentially abnormal tissue within its structure. This creates a potential weak spot. Guess where abnormal stress and strain are likely to show up again in the future? You got it. At those "weak" spots. So, ideally, surgery should be avoided unless it is the last resort.

If somebody says, "Let's try surgery", that probably isn't the best course of action. Once you start doing any kind of invasive procedures to your elbow, you start getting scar tissue building up. Nerves can become impinged within the scar tissue. Your elbow will never be the same again. It can't be because there's scar tissue in there that wasn't there before. If you heal it, non-surgically and non-invasively, your elbow can be as good as it was before.

Every conservative form of treatment should be investigated before undergoing surgery, and that is true for any issue. It's upsetting for people to believe that having surgery will cure them and when they wake up, they are still feeling symptoms. Many clients who find me have been disappointed in this way and are astounded when a non-invasive approach works better for them. Surgery is not a panacea. However, the treatment protocol you're going to learn in this book reverses the damage to the tendon, which allows the tendon to recover. You'll learn how to do this safely in chapter 9.

6. You've got it for life, there's nothing you can do, you'll just have to live with it and take pain pills

Mythbuster: Green et al (2002) showed that *"NSAIDS can be effective initially, but not in the long term."* This fits with the acute inflammatory model, which resolves over a short period of time - more on this later.

Do you want to keep managing episodic elbow pain over time because it will keep coming back or do you want to get rid of it once and for all? Most people say, "I want to get rid of it for good." That is the recognition of not just getting to the point of being pain-free, but additionally what else needs to be done to heal the tendon, so the pain will not return. Essentially, you can get yourself to the pain-free point if you do not use your arm. You rest the tendon and the symptoms settle down. Great, you think to yourself, I am cured! But hold on, the tendon is still injured and will likely let you know as soon as you try to lift your cup of coffee with that arm again.

If you take an ultrasound scan of an affected tendon, often the tendon looks thickened, compared to a normal tendon.[7] This is due to the pathology of tennis elbow. Resting it, or using basic therapies, can allow the irritated tendon to start to feel better. But even if a patient feels pain-free, the ultrasound scan would reveal no change in the appearance of the tendon. It would still look the same as it did at the height of the problem. Therefore, the symptoms can keep coming back because the underlying pathology has not changed. Some treatments reverse this pathology. The tendon returns to normal. You will learn how to do this later in the book.

Regarding "There's nothing you can do to help it". There's always something you can do, but guidance to ensure you are doing the correct things at the correct time is paramount. Is it easy? Not always, but it sure beats years of discomfort and declining activity. I've heard of people who have suffered with tennis elbow for as long as 30 years. In fact, two of the sufferers I spoke with recently were in that category.

There are small changes that can be made, but you must be ready to make those changes. I have made suggestions to people in the past and have been met with resistance because they didn't want to make changes, or, better said, they didn't believe that small changes would make any difference, so they weren't willing to try. Doing nothing will never result in elbow pain completely resolving. It will always come back, most likely more intensely and for longer each time.

"You'll have to take pain pills for the rest of your life." This action leads to wasted time, money, and energy, not to mention the negative effects this can have on your body such as nausea, weakness, and a weakened immune system.[8] Many people are thrilled to find that this statement is just not true. Pain pills are not good for your internal organs and being dependent on chemicals such as these is draining. There are many different options for pain relief - you can explore these in chapter 6.

7. You only get it in your dominant arm... but then it will spread to the other arm

Mythbuster: Many golfers experience tennis elbow in their non-dominant arm.

Usually, people get tennis elbow in their dominant arm, due to repetitive motion and/or unaccustomed activities. However, I have seen many golfers who get tennis elbow, not golfer's elbow, but tennis elbow in their non-dominant arm. This has to do with the biomechanics of the swing, the way they're gripping the club or just straight overuse. For example, I helped a lady who had developed tennis elbow in her non-dominant arm, from playing lots of golf once she retired. You'll be happy to hear that she is back on the golf course and 100% pain-free.

It could be that you are renovating your house and suddenly, you're spending hours and hours laying patio stones or with an electric drill in your hands. Maybe you irritate your non-dominant side because it's not used to doing the things you are asking it to do. One client had been frantically cleaning her house before relatives came over for the holidays and she got tennis elbow in her nondominant arm because it wasn't used to doing so much activity all at once.

Either side can be affected, or even both sides. If someone delays getting the correct treatment, then unfortunately it is possible to develop similar symptoms in the other arm too. The sooner you start doing the correct treatment, the sooner the symptoms resolve and the less likely they are to affect other structures. The longer you feel it, the more structures can be affected, and this may lead to the other side developing issues too.

If you're right-handed and you're using your right hand all the time for whatever repetitive motion it may be, and you develop tennis elbow. Guess what, you're not going to want to use that arm because now it hurts. You'll likely take over those repetitive motions with the other arm and you can irritate the other side from that action. It can be a compensatory mechanism.

People who have suffered for a longer time tend to have abnormalities in their shoulder and neck that can affect all the soft tissues of those areas too. It shouldn't be lost on you that some pretty major soft tissues are coming out of the neck, passing by the shoulders, and down the arms – the nerves. It is extremely common for the nerves to become involved in someone suffering from prolonged tennis elbow symptoms.

Imagine the nervous system as one continuous structure, from your brain, down your spinal cord with nerves exiting the spine at every single level. As one vertebra sits on top of another, there are small holes on either side of the spine where the nerves come out and these nerves travel down to the tips of your fingers or the tips of your toes, depending on which level they have exited from. It seems logical to think that if the nerve on one side becomes irritated due to tennis elbow pathology, then it could affect the same nerve on the other side of the body. Hence symptoms can appear on the other side.

Let me put that another way, tennis elbow is a tendon problem. Tendon problems appear to be closely correlated to nerve problems. The nerves come out of the neck and go down the arm and there are similar nerves that go down the other arm. If you irritate a tendon and a nerve that's close to it, on one side, it becomes more likely that you will irritate a tendon somewhere else. Now it might not be tennis elbow. It might be golfer's elbow, a problem on the inside of the elbow. It might be a shoulder tendon. It might be a foot tendon or a knee tendon, but if you have a tendon issue, many times a nerve is involved in some way. The nervous system becomes hyper-sensitized. This is the big picture that many healthcare professionals miss. Most of the time when people have suffered with tennis elbow for longer than 3 months, a nerve will become irritated and if the nervous system becomes hypersensitized, other tendons can easily become affected too. You'll learn more about this concept later in the book.

8. Tennis elbow is inflammation

Mythbuster: Buchanan et al (2022) described tennis elbow as *"demonstrating a notable lack of traditional inflammatory cells (macrophages, lymphocytes, neutrophils) within the tissue."*

I guess that this myth-buster just blew your mind. Am I right? To investigate this myth, we must first understand how the healing process takes place. The healing process can be broken down into 3 distinct phases: the inflammation phase (the first 7 days after an injury), the repair phase (between 4 days and 2 months duration), and the remodeling phase (6 weeks to 12 months).[9, 10]

If the symptoms have been present for longer than a week, there are likely to be few inflammatory cells in or around the tendon. The way anti-inflammatory pills work is by reducing inflammation, which in turn decreases symptoms, and you feel better. So, if there are no inflammatory cells, there is nothing for the anti-inflammatory pills to work on and so your symptoms remain unchanged.

However, using this understanding of different phases of the healing process, it is possible to utilize anti-inflammatory medications in the event of an acute flare-up. For example, if you bump your elbow on a door frame, this could elicit swelling and bruising, which is a typical acute inflammatory response. Anti-inflammatories can work in the early phases, and they can also work if you flare up by doing something out of the ordinary. If someone had been experiencing tennis elbow symptoms for 12 months, we would recognize them to be in the remodeling phase of healing. However, if they were to undertake an unusual activity, such as moving to a new house; the heavy lifting, repeated motions, and consistent gripping of this activity may well irritate the tendon enough to cause an acute inflammation on top of the chronic problem. A new injury on top of an old one, if you like. This could potentially be a good opportunity for an anti-inflammatory medication to help reduce symptoms, as the acute phase of healing has been rekindled. You'll learn how to treat these situations in chapter 6.

To sum up, if you are in the very early stages of tennis elbow, meaning you've had symptoms for a few days, anti-inflammatories may help your symptoms. If you've had this for three months, three years, or longer, anti-inflammatories are probably not going to make a whole lot of difference. When you have a soft tissue injury, the initial response is that the body sends inflammatory cells to the injured area to start the healing process. If the inflammatory cells are there, anti-inflammatory medication can work on them and help to settle things down, but if you have had this for longer, you are way past that initial phase of the healing process and so there are probably very few inflammatory cells there for the anti-inflammatory medication to work on.

Inflammation is the body's natural response to injury, and it has a set time frame. After 12 weeks, the inflammatory phase is well and truly over. So, why do some people still experience symptoms after 3 months? The concept of chronic pain[11] has been around for many years now, but we still have much to learn. What we do know is that when someone is still experiencing pain 3 months after an injury, or has symptoms that last longer than 12 weeks, the nervous system has become hypersensitized. This phenomenon can be resolved with targeted treatment. A skilled therapist can identify the causes of the symptoms that are still being felt. Often, this key part is missing from rehab and so people don't get better. You'll learn more about this concept in greater detail later in the book.

9. It's your age

Mythbuster: I've helped teenagers who had tennis elbow.

Tennis elbow is not a condition due to age. Granted, we do heal faster the younger we are, but tennis elbow isn't specifically an age-related problem. It's a degeneration of the tendon, but not an aged-related degeneration like osteoarthritis which is the wear and tear of the joints that everyone tends to get as we age. To explain this, we need to back up a bit and learn about the anatomy of the area. A tendon is a connective tissue that attaches a muscle to the bone. That's all a tendon is. But, if a tendon becomes overworked, it will start to break down, that is, degenerate. This degeneration of the tendon has nothing to do with age though. Athletes and kids can get tennis elbow if they overuse the tendon enough.

To give you a visualization of what happens during the degeneration of the tendon, imagine a tightly wound rope. This is what a normal tendon would look like on an ultrasound scan. An ultrasound scan is different from ultrasound treatment that you may have heard about or even experienced. An ultrasound scan is the imaging they do for pregnant ladies when they see the baby. An ultrasound scan can be performed on soft tissues, such as those around the elbow so that the tissues can be seen.

If you did an ultrasound scan of a normal tendon, that tendon should look like a rope. All the fibers are very uniform, packed tightly together, and they are all in the same direction. On an ultrasound scan of a tennis elbow, imagine that rope-like tendon unraveling. The fibers are no longer uniform or packed tightly together, but they are separated and haphazard. Cells can get in between the fibers, where they are not supposed to be, and cause irritation, weakness, and other symptoms. That's what a degenerated tendon, or a tennis elbow tendon, looks like on an ultrasound scan.

Despite this sounding dramatic, there is good news. Recent developments in treatment techniques have resulted in much higher percentages of symptoms completely resolving. The ultrasound scans of these patients also show a reversal of the degeneration process.[12] It is not often that we can say that an issue can be reversed and resolved, but this is one of those times.

To have elbow pain is not just part of aging. It's not something that anybody should have to put up with or experience. Many people experience episodic elbow pain and think there's nothing they can do. They experience a flare-up of pain and it settles down. The next time it comes back, it's a little bit worse, but it'll settle down. The next time it comes back, it's a little bit worse again, it takes a little bit longer to settle down and then it'll settle down. The next time it comes back...etc. People get stuck in this cycle. The symptoms can settle down, but if you don't do the correct things at the correct time to heal the tendon, it will keep coming back. That's why I stress to people that once they've got rid of the pain, if they don't do the other things that they need to do, like correct the movement patterns, get muscles stronger than they are right now, and stretch things out that are tight, it will keep coming back. Keep reading.

10. Your parents had it, and so will you

Mythbuster: Alakhdar Mohmara et al (2020) found *"the genotype for SNP COL11A1 rs3753841 was associated with elbow tendon pathology. However, significant relationships were also found between the anthropometric variables; BMI, percent body fat, waist circumference, and elbow tendon pathology."*

Basically, genetics can play a part in elbow pain, but many things can affect it too. For example, my Grandad had a total knee replacement, and my Dad has also had a total knee replacement. Now that I know I have a genetic predisposition to osteoarthritis of the knees; I can take care of my knees.

I just completed my second marathon. Notice I said 'completed'. I didn't say 'ran' my second marathon. I know I can complete 26.2 miles if I use a combination of running and walking. If I try to run the whole way, I can only get to 10K (6 miles) before my knees start to tell me I'm going too far. Using that knowledge, I can modify my activity to preserve my knees but still participate in activities I love to do.

As specified by the research in the mythbuster, maintaining a healthy body weight and the associated factors that go along with it, were seen to help decrease the likelihood of pathology occurring in the participants who had the genetic predisposition. Indeed, Vaquero-Picado et al (2017) found *"smoking and obesity to be significant risk factors for experiencing tennis elbow."*

11. You need an X-ray or an MRI scan to see what's wrong

Mythbuster: Speers et al (2018) stated *"lateral elbow tendinosis is a clinical diagnosis and therefore radiological investigation is seldom required and reserved for those who fail to improve."*

Tennis elbow can be diagnosed by performing clinical tests and doesn't need imaging. Imaging for the elbow generally involves X-rays, MRI scans, and maybe ultrasound scans. Are these procedures necessary for most people with elbow pain? No. So, why do many people get irradiated, if it's not necessary? Surely, the doctor needs to see what's wrong with your elbow? No, as the mythbuster stated, tennis elbow is a diagnosis that can be made from clinical testing and judgment. Imaging is rarely needed to make this diagnosis.

If you have had an x-ray, what did it show? Degeneration, bone spurs, joint disease. Those are some scary words right there. But what do they mean? And is that what is causing your pain?

X-rays only show the bones. Therefore, unless you have a fracture in a bone, all the soft tissues; muscles, tendons, ligaments, and nerves, don't show up on x-rays. Most people have no identifiable cause for their pain on an x-ray.[13] Let's avoid unnecessary costs and radiation.

If you've had an MRI, what did it show? Degeneration, tendonitis, tears, effusion. But is that what is causing your elbow pain? MRIs are great because they show everything. MRIs are also not great because they show everything. MRI scans do show the soft tissues, but in most cases, the result of the MRI scan isn't going to change the treatment needed to resolve the cause of the problem. In fact, Savnik et al, (2004) showed *"MRI scans demonstrate an altered signal around the lateral epicondyle in just 2/3 of patients with a tennis elbow diagnosis."* MRIs are also costly and some people struggle with claustrophobia or panic attacks due to the confined nature of the procedure itself. Do you need an MRI to confirm your diagnosis? No. Clinical tests that your doctor or physical therapist can do will be sufficient to determine which structures are causing your symptoms.

Most elbow pain is due to damage to soft tissues, rather than the bones. All tissues can heal over time. However, as previously mentioned, it's important to be doing the right things at the right time, to get the right result. Unfortunately, most people don't do the right things at the right time to achieve optimal healing and so set themselves up for recurring symptoms. If you do the right things, you stretch and strengthen your elbow, you can become pain-free, despite what your MRI or x-ray may show.

12. Exercise will make it worse and you're in too much pain to come to therapy

Mythbuster: The right exercise at the right time won't make you worse and will make you better. Therapy should NOT make you worse.

But do the wrong exercise and you may well increase your symptoms. Equally, doing the right exercise but at the wrong time can also make things worse. This can happen when you search the internet for exercises to treat tennis elbow.

Please attend your therapy sessions especially if you are struggling. Therapy should not hurt you, and if it does, something is not right. There are many different strategies for pain relief. It can even be super helpful to attend therapy when you are in pain, so that the therapist can identify exactly what is causing the problem and then administer treatment techniques for immediate relief and advise you on what to do, and not do, at home as well.

13. Physical therapy (physiotherapy) doesn't work for tennis elbow

Mythbuster: Let's look at a couple of myths in combination: Coombes et al (2013) showed that *"physiotherapy was effective in treating unilateral lateral epicondylalgia"*, however, they also showed that *"administering a steroid injection negated the positive effects of physiotherapy."*

So basically, if you are sent for physical therapy, it CAN help. But, if you have a steroid shot too, it won't...because of the steroid shot! How many well-meaning doctors are setting their patients up to fail by trying to help them with steroid injections?

When I hear people say they have tennis elbow and have tried physical therapy and it didn't work, it makes me sad. Physical therapy does work, but only if you are doing the right things at the right time. The thousands of clients I've helped are a testament to that. Physical therapy does work when it's done in the way it needs to be done. However, the issue is that not all physical therapy is the same. Let me explain.

For years, tennis elbow was treated as a standard soft tissue injury. Physical therapy encompasses many different treatment modalities and in the past, many of these were quite passive. Think electrotherapy, ultrasound treatment, electrical stimulation, laser, massage therapy, or other soft tissue techniques. Basically, the therapist was doing things to the patient. The patient was not an active participant in the treatment, they were passive.

Therapy would focus only on the involved elbow and about 50% of patients would recover from that episode. The 50% that didn't get better would go on to have surgery and then 50% of them would improve. 50% would not. There were many "returners" to therapy, as the elbow would periodically flare up. Thankfully, now those numbers can look very different. Many of the passive treatments are ineffective in healing tennis elbow; Dingemanse et al, (2014) showed *"no conclusive evidence that any electrotherapy modality is effective at healing lateral epicondylitis."*

However, active treatments, such as strengthening (and a very specific form of strengthening that you'll learn in chapter 9) are incredibly effective at resolving tennis elbow. Every single person can make a full recovery and return to everything they want to be doing, with no restrictions, but only if they do exactly what they need to do at the correct time. Individual guidance is essential.

Not all clinics are created equally. Many patients have experienced therapy, where they were one of many people in a big room. Where the therapist would spend a few minutes with them before they were passed onto an unlicensed aide. Or were literally on a treatment conveyor belt, moving from one spot for heat to another spot for stretching, then electrical stimulation or ultrasound, and then ice. They would get the same treatment every time and the same treatment as everyone else. There was no individualization, no change in treatment plan depending on the patient's symptoms and no progression to ensure the problem didn't return. I apologize to these patients, and I apologize to you if you have experienced this subpar version of therapy. How many people have experienced this and thought to themselves that physical therapy didn't work, so I must need surgery? It's my mission to save people from this fate.

Would you go and see your primary care physician for an operation to repair a hole in your heart? No? Me neither. I'd want to go and see a cardiac specialist surgeon, preferably one who only does the procedure I needed. The point I'm trying to get across here is that there is a huge difference between generalists and specialists. Most people know that medical doctors have different specializations, but did you know that that is also the case among many healthcare professions?

You may have been sent to the local general physical therapy clinic by your insurance or your family doctor when you needed some therapy. All PT is the same, right? Wrong. Just like specialist surgeons who have trained for years and then honed their skills during residencies and fellowships, on continuing education courses, and under the guidance of mentors, physical therapists have too.

Physical therapists are not all the same. I have colleagues who are specialist physical therapists in the treatment of lymphedema. They work with cancer patients. Some physical therapists work in pediatrics. They work with kids. Some physical therapists work in women's health, such as pelvic floor issues.

Whenever you have any kind of issue, you want to find a specialist for that particular issue. That is a reason general physical therapy doesn't work for tennis elbow. General therapists only see one or two tennis elbow sufferers a year. They haven't got enough experience in healing tennis elbow. It's not their fault. They're busy treating all the backs, necks, knees, shoulders, and everything else that comes through the door. But if you really want to get down to the core of the problem that you have and heal it properly, you need to work with a specialist.

Physical therapy does work hands down. You've just got to find the right therapist. That's why I recommend seeking an experienced physical therapist who specializes in treating tennis elbow. It does everyone a disservice if the therapist doesn't fully understand the complexity of the issue and how many different structures are potentially contributing to the symptoms. You can't just focus treatment on the elbow alone as that strategy doesn't work. Unless all of the contributing structures are addressed the issue will definitely return or the poor patient will never feel relief in the first place, neither of which is an acceptable outcome.

Specialists are naturally more skilled in their particular field than their generalist peers. If you have tennis elbow, wouldn't you want to see the top specialist in that field? Someone who only helps people who have the same problem as you. A specialist will likely spend all their time working with clients like you. A generalist may see someone with a problem like yours, but then they see someone with a neck issue, the next patient has a knee injury, and then a sprained ankle comes hobbling in. So, if you're looking for somebody who can help get you to the end destination of actually healing, not just get you pain-free, you've found the answer here in your hands.

14. Virtual treatment won't work for tennis elbow

Mythbuster: Janela et al (2022) studied this conept and found *"The significant improvement observed in clinical outcomes, alongside high engagement, and satisfaction suggests patient acceptance of this care delivery mode."*

Physical therapy is now a possibility due to technology and virtual visits. "How can you do physical therapy virtually? Don't you need to touch me?" This is a common misconception, not just among clients, but within the physical therapy community too. When COVID-19 caused lockdowns around the world many physical therapy clinics closed their doors. When lockdown closed my physical clinic location, we immediately transitioned everyone to virtual visits. No one went without treatment. We actually added services to keep our community healthy, boost immunity, and prevent morbidity.

We have successfully rehabbed post-surgical clients, helped clients regain their mobility and independence, resolved ergonomic issues related to working from home, continued classes, and added courses, all in the digital environment. We have helped more people, in more countries than ever before and our results are equivalent to my in-person results.

Most people can find relief after just one session, so, why then do people not do that? They are skeptical, I get it. When you've been let down by so many things you've tried before, you get to the point where you think nothing will work for you. You don't want to waste any more time and money on something else that will let you down. It's completely understandable. That's why a great strategy can be to search for success stories from people just like you. You can find many of my clients' success stories sprinkled throughout this book.

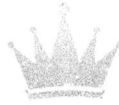

CHAPTER 2

What Is Tennis Elbow?

The sub-heading here would be "When an 'itis' isn't inflammation". The term "tennis elbow" doesn't have "itis" in it, but lateral epicondylitis is the medical terminology for tennis elbow. "-itis" means inflammation in Greek. In Chapter 1, you learned that anti-inflammatories don't often work on tennis elbow, or lateral epicondylitis, and the reason for that is because the inflammatory response, the inflammation, the "itis", only occurs in the very early stage of the condition. Once you get beyond the first three weeks, there is not much inflammation there[9, 10] unless you've irritated it. So, lateral epicondylitis is not a good descriptive name for this problem, unless you've had it for a very short time, or have recently irritated it, in which case it would apply.

You may hear the term lateral epicondylopathy; meaning lateral (on the outside), epicondyl- (the bony bit of the elbow), -opathy, which means pathology. Essentially, there is a pathology on the outside of your elbow. This is an umbrella term because we don't know if it's an "itis" or something else. You may have heard the term "tendinosis". "Itis" means acute inflammation or a problem that you've not had for very long. "Osis'" means chronic or a problem hanging around for a while. "Tendinopathy" covers everything.

Let's dive into the anatomy. Firstly, let's consider the bones. The long bone that comes down from the shoulder to the elbow is called the humerus. Two bones create your forearm, the radius, and the ulna. The lateral epicondyle is the bony point on the outside of the elbow, likely where it's tender. This is where the common extensor tendon attaches. This is the tendon that is affected by tennis elbow. The common extensor tendon attaches the muscles of the forearm to the lateral epicondyle part of the bone. When the muscles switch on, they lift the hand up at the wrist and the tendon takes force through it. A tendon is basically a connective tissue. Tendons attach muscles to bones.

In tennis elbow, the tendon is affected. In the very early stages of this problem, the first few days, you might have some inflammation. After that, you likely don't have much, unless you irritate it specifically. Why then, do you still feel pain? Great question. The answer is that the tendon is degenerating. This is a degeneration that has nothing to do with age. The word "degeneration", can conjure up images of falling apart. It's all to do with the pathology and that's what irritates the tendon.

Connell et al (2001) remarked *"Using ultrasound scans, a normal tendon is recognized as parallel-arranged fibrils without disruption. When degenerative tendinopathy is present, there is heterogeneous thickening of the tendon with areas of decreased echogenicity."* All that to say a normal tendon looks like a tightly wound rope. A tendon affected by tennis elbow looks like someone twisted the rope the wrong way, so the fibers splayed apart.

The reason that tennis elbow can last so long is that tendons have an extremely poor blood supply. In the picture, you can see the muscle is shaded in. Muscles have a great blood supply because they need lots of oxygen to let them work and move. Tendons, as you can see in the picture, are shaded white as they don't have a good blood supply. A tendon is essentially a connective tissue that attaches muscle to the bone. So, it doesn't need a lot of blood supply to do that job. However, it does need a good blood supply to heal and tendons don't have a good blood supply and that's the reason they take so long to heal. Therefore, we want to increase the circulation to the area. The body is amazing. The body recognizes that it needs to get more blood flowing into the tendon to heal it. So, the body grows new blood vessels into the tendon to try and get more blood to it. However, this is not normal. The tendon shouldn't have these new blood vessels in it. And it turns out these new blood vessels struggle to do a good job anyway.

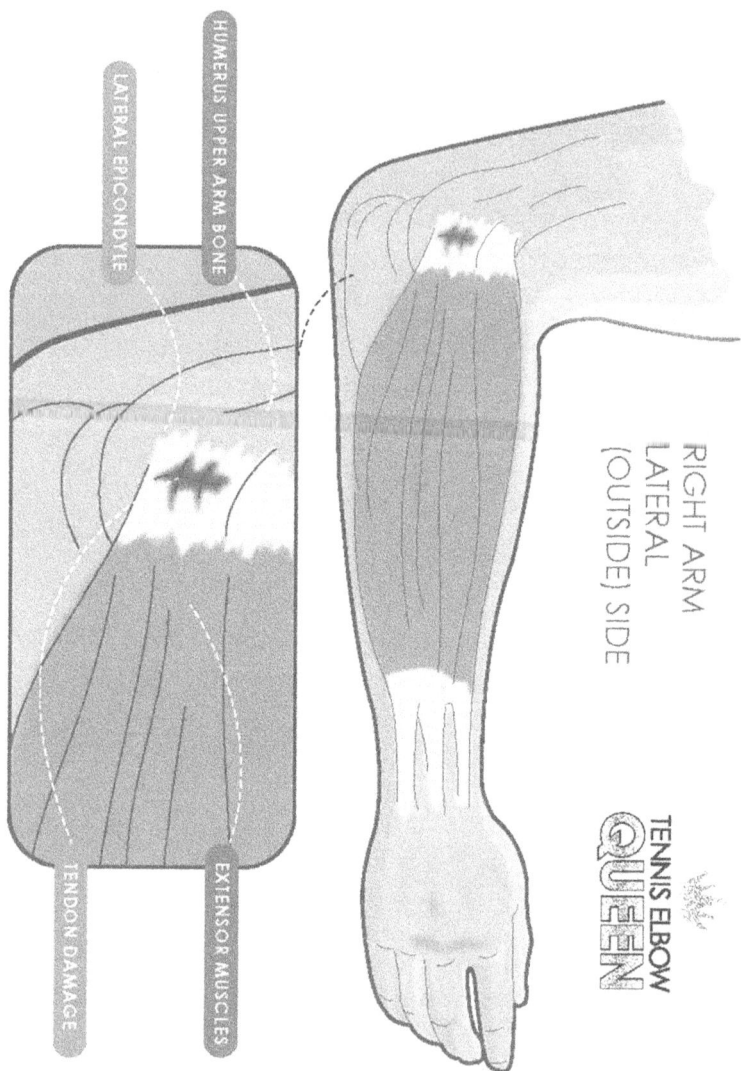

LATERAL EPICONDYLE

HUMERUS UPPER ARM BONE

TENDON DAMAGE

EXTENSOR MUSCLES

RIGHT ARM
LATERAL
(OUTSIDE) SIDE

TENNIS ELBOW
QUEEN

As previously mentioned ultrasound scans can view the tendon. There is also a type of ultrasound scan that can view blood vessels. Therefore, if these additional blood vessels are seen on an ultrasound scan as well, it's part of the pathology and is called neovascularization; "neo" means new, and "vascularization" means blood vessels.[23]

But how does that happen to the tissues?

Bazancir et al, 2019 hypothesized that *"the tensile response may be the responsible mechanism in the pathophysiology of lateral epicondylitis due to the microanatomy of the extensor carpi radialis brevis (ECRB) muscle and its functioning in the elongated position. An elongated position leads to elongation of the sarcomere length by forming a functional traction angle in the ECRB muscle. The elongated sarcomere length negatively affects muscular microcirculation. Poor microcirculation triggers ischemia in the muscle and tendon and leads to an increase in immature Type III collagen synthesis. Disruption of the collagen continuity and the loss of load-bearing capacity initiate the neovascularization process. This situation accelerates the degeneration process in the tendon and prevents healing."*

Wow!

All that means is that because the muscle tends to work in a lengthened or stretched-out position, this decreases the circulation within the muscle. This causes the muscle and tendon to break down and it struggles to heal while this is going on. This is why you have to stop this negative cycle to heal. If you don't change what you are doing, the tissues can't heal. It's as simple as that. Something has to change.

Did you notice the word "neovascularization" above? It means "new blood vessels". Järvinen (2020) expanded on this by stating *"tendons respond to hypoxia by secreting angiogenic growth factors that induce the growth of neovessels (new vessels) in tendinopathy. These neovessels are hyperpermeable; they leak and do not have proper perfusion, failing to deliver oxygen and nutrients required for tissue regeneration. Fibrin-rich exudates leak from the neovessels, which results in fibrinoid degeneration, a typical feature of tendinosis in tendinopathy."*

Phew! So, while the body is trying to help the healing process by growing new blood vessels, unfortunately, they leak and actually irritate the injury. While this is something that tissue engineers are contemplating, there are certain simple strategies that you can employ that will maximize the healing of your tissues in this context. You'll find them in chapter 6.

Years ago, basic therapies were used to treat tennis elbow and about half of patients would feel better afterwards. However, if you did an ultrasound scan of their elbow, the tendon would still look degenerated. The tendon did not change. Symptoms settled down, so the patient felt better, but it didn't truly heal and that's why symptoms would return because the tendon was still degenerated.

Thankfully, we've known about more effective types of treatment techniques for over 20 years. With these newer ways of healing tendons, essentially, you don't just settle the symptoms, you improve the tendon. If you did an ultrasound scan of that elbow once it is healed, imagine seeing that rope tightened back up again as it should be. The thickened injured tendon returns to a more normal size.[24] It's truly amazing what the body can do. It can heal itself with the right environment, and by doing the right things at the right time.

Why it can last so long

Why do some people suffer with this for such a long time if we know that tennis elbow can be completely resolved? If somebody has had tennis elbow for several years, not only is it affecting the tendon, but it will be affecting other structures too. It's like a ripple effect. If you drop a pebble into a pond, the ripples spread out over time. If the elbow is where your problem started, the longer you have it, the further the ripple effect is going to spread. It can affect the forearm muscles and your wrist and hand. It can affect the biceps muscle, the shoulder joint, your shoulder blade and neck.

The longer you've had tennis elbow, the more tissues are involved and they all need addressing because they will not be functioning correctly. They will not be receiving their normal neural input, which is messages from the nerves. They're not getting the correct messages from the nerves because the pathology has been going on for a long time. This can all be resolved too, but it needs addressing for you to heal. This issue is often not addressed.

If you go to see somebody and say, "I have tennis elbow, I've had it for three years" and they say, "Let me look at your elbow". Okay, that's a great start and can confirm the diagnosis, but that's likely not the whole story. If you just focus treatment on the elbow and don't work on everything else that has been affected by the prolonged tennis elbow, the issue will come back every time. Unfortunately, that's why people say treatment failed them. Everything needs to be addressed and then it can be resolved once and for all so that it does not come back, and you can do everything you want to do with no restrictions whatsoever.

Xu et al (2023) noted that *"lateral epicondylitis is a common clinical disease characterized by lateral elbow pain,* **seriously affecting patients' daily life and work."** Non-sufferers have no idea how painful this condition can be. It's not unusual to hear from clients how their issue has been trivialized by co-workers, friends, or even family members. "What are you moaning about? It's just tennis elbow!" clients have been told when they can't do simple daily activities because their elbow hurts too much.

Where are you on the pain phase scale described by Nirschl (2015)

Nirschl pain phase scale for athletic overuse injuries

Phase 1	Stiffness or mild soreness after activity, usually gone within 24 hours
Phase 2	Stiffness or mild soreness before activity that is relieved by a warm-up. Symptoms are not present during activity but return after, lasting up to 48 hours
Phase 3	Stiffness or mild soreness before specific sport or occupational activity. Pain is partially relieved by warm-up. It is minimally present during activity but does not cause the athlete to alter their activity
Phase 4	Pain is similar to but more intense than phase 3 pain. Phase 4 pain causes the athlete to alter the performance of the activity. Mild pain may also be noticed with activities of daily living
Phase 5	Significant (moderate or greater) pain before, during, and after activity, causing alteration of activity. Pain occurs with activities of daily living but does not cause a major change in them
Phase 6	Phase 5 pain that persists even with complete rest. Phase 6 pain disrupts simple activities of daily living and prohibits doing household chores
Phase 7	Phase 6 pain that also disrupts sleep consistently. Pain is aching in nature and intensifies with activity

The higher the phase you're in, the more structures are likely affected and they are likely more severely affected. Note the phase you are in and today's date here:

Phase number:

Date:

What is pain?

Pain is a sensation perceived in the brain. It can indicate tissue damage, for example picking up a hot pan. OW! Your brain perceives the intense heat through your tissues and sends a message down to your hand to "let go". But does pain always mean tissue damage? No, not always. Try this out, right now; pull your little finger back as far as it can go. Now push it just a little further. OW! Your body is warning you to not push any further, or tissue damage will happen. This is a protective mechanism.

Then, if I'm feeling pain, I shouldn't push through, right? As in a few answers I give, it depends. If you've just injured yourself, as in it's really recent, within 3 days, then "No", you shouldn't push it. But if you were injured over 3 months ago, then you are safer to push. A Licensed Physical Therapist can guide you through this situation. Their knowledge of tissue healing at particular time frames will allow them to make the best selection of treatment options at each particular stage.

Chronic pain

Chronic pain is a situation that can develop after someone has been feeling pain for over 3 months. Not everyone develops chronic pain, and it's not known why some people do and some people don't. More is being learned about chronic pain all the time.

Chronic pain is real. Not that long ago, people who suffered from chronic pain were told that it was all in their heads. Ironically, to a degree, that is true, as when chronic pain occurs, there are physiological and anatomical changes in the brain.[25] Chronic pain is a cycle that leads the nervous system to become hypersensitized.[26] This is called central sensitization and means that it doesn't take much to trigger a nerve. Let me explain that a little further.

All nerves are stimulated by certain sensations, for example, touch. When does a firm touch, such as a handshake, become painful like a pinch? Your nervous system delivers the information on how hard, or soft, the pressure is. Now imagine your nervous system is hypersensitized, and that firm handshake feels like a pinch. OW. The nervous system is sending too many messages, too quickly, and the person feels way more than they should due to the level of pressure being applied.

Thankfully, there are treatment techniques that can normalize the nervous system. This is one of the most common missing links in the treatment of tennis elbow. 95% of the tennis elbow clients I see have some sort of nerve involvement as part of their problem. Be sure to ask your healthcare provider about how they will address the issue of the hypersensitized nervous system. In my experience, if the nervous system is not addressed correctly, the problem cannot truly be resolved and will return.

This is why I added Empowered Relief® to the comprehensive program. Empowered Relief® is an evidence-based, single-session pain class that rapidly equips attendees with pain management skills. It was developed by pain psychology doctors at Stanford University and they have spent over 10 years researching it's effectiveness. From the comfort of your home, it takes just two hours to learn simple yet impactful strategies that you can use right away to manage your chronic pain.

Empowered Relief® is taught exclusively by certified instructors. This live, virtual class helps people address ongoing pain that interferes with their quality of life. Research shows that attendees experience lasting benefits from Empowered Relief®, including reduced pain intensity, better sleep, lower stress, and more.

You will walk away from the 2-hour training with:

- A deeper understanding of the neuroscience behind pain
- A robust set of skills that you can count on to decrease the ways chronic pain negatively affects your daily life
- An audio file combining binaural beats with guided meditation
- An individualized plan you can turn to for pain relief

If persistent pain gets in the way of living the life you want, I hope you will join me for my next Empowered Relief® class. Learn more and sign up here:

https://www.tenniselbowqueen.com/empoweredrelief

How do you know if you have nerve involvement? What do nerve symptoms feel like? Pain, electric shocks, tingling, pins and needles, numbness, ants crawling on the skin, water trickling; clients have used all these descriptions. I had a new client recently describe "knives" in her arm. Can you relate to some of these symptoms?

What causes it? Several different problems can cause nerve symptoms, so what works for one person, may not work for another if the cause of their symptoms is different. Nerve symptoms can be caused by pressure on the nerve from an internal structure such as a bulging or herniated disc in the spine, an inflamed or arthritic joint in the neck, a tight muscle in the shoulder or forearm, pressure on the nerve from an external source like a hard table or armrest or shortening of the nerve due to a muscle imbalance or not using the arm normally. As you can see, there's a lot to investigate with nerve symptoms, which an experienced practitioner can test and talk you through.

The nerve itself can become irritated. A nerve is a soft tissue like a muscle or a ligament. Soft tissues can shorten and tighten. They adapt to the stresses and strains that are put through them. For example, if you've not stretched out your pecs for a long time and you do lots of work on building up those muscles but don't stretch them out, they'll get tight. Similarly, if you don't stretch a nerve out, or you're not mobilizing a nerve, it can become tight, and you can get tension within the nerve itself that can then become irritated and uncomfortable.

Jalovaara et al (1989) found that *"30% of tennis elbow sufferers were actually suffering from radial tunnel syndrome."* Bonczar et al (2023) found that *"over 40% of patients had more than one source of lateral elbow pain, with 35% having posterior interosseous nerve entrapment."*

In my experience, over 95% of the clients I see with a diagnosis of tennis elbow have some kind of concurrent nerve issue. It's essential to treat the nerve. If that is not addressed then you won't find relief. That's why my method works on the nervous system from day 1. If you haven't found help yet, despite trying EVERYTHING, it's likely this is the missing piece.

Why do anything about a bit of a niggle?

Why do people have this problem when they shouldn't? People put things off. We're all guilty of it. Guess how long it took me to write this book? Sometimes when we put things off, it can have a detrimental effect on us and our quality of life. If someone went to see a Licensed Physical Therapist, with a bit of a niggle in their elbow, it would be pretty straightforward to figure out what would be the best course of action for that person, get them doing the right things, prevent it from getting worse and alleviate it.

Unfortunately, that rarely happens. Most people wait until they can't take it any longer or are unable to pick up the crying baby, or until the pain has them sobbing to their spouse at 3 a.m., or when the nerve pressure becomes nerve damage, and they lose their strength. Guess how much longer these issues take to resolve? So much longer. However, that's human nature, we put things off until we have to deal with them. If you have a bit of a niggle at the moment, do yourself a favor and get it looked at now. Imagine the heartache, pain, time, energy, and money you'll be saving yourself and your family.

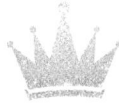

CHAPTER 3

What Causes Tennis Elbow?

Why did you get tennis elbow? There are a few different reasons identified in this chapter:

- Overuse
- Altered biomechanics
- Direct trauma
- Compensation mechanism
- Antibiotics
- Ergonomics
- Central sensitization

Research shows that:

- 1–3% of the population will suffer from tennis elbow (Karabinov et al, 2022)
- 50% of tennis players will experience tennis elbow at some point in their playing career (Cutts et al, 2019)
- 26% of manual laborers will develop tennis elbow (Park et al, 2021)
- Overuse is the number one cause (Buchanan et al, 2022)
- Chronic pain starts after three months of symptoms (Raffaeli et al, 2021)

- Herquelot et al (2013) found *"no significant difference between the incidence of tennis elbow in men and women."* They also found *"workers aged >45 years had a higher incidence than those aged <30 years."* So, if you're a manual laborer, between the ages of 30 and 45, who enjoys playing tennis – you're reading the right book!

Has this ever happened to you? You wake up one sunny morning and spring out of bed, ready to enjoy the day, when BAM. Suddenly, you are hit with the pain on the outside of your elbow. What is going on? Is it serious? What should you do? You cross to the bathroom and search around the medicine cabinet for some anti-inflammatories or painkillers. You hate taking pills, but this pain is so bad. But which pills should you take? You're not sure, so you start trying to read the tiny writing on the side of the bottle, while the pain seems to be spreading down your arm. Then, you give in on trying to read the label and take two pain pills. That's got to be OK, right?

You look at your reflection in the mirror and don't recognize the face contorted with agony. As you look over your shoulder in the mirror, your gaze rests on the shower. A nice hot shower. That'll work, won't it? Wait, should you be using heat or ice? Why oh, why is this so hard? You forgo the shower and head into the kitchen to make your coffee. As you do so, you reach out to pick up your favorite mug. OUCH! That was not a good idea as the pain is now down through your forearm. Oh, when will the pain pills kick in? This pain is so bad, there must be something seriously wrong, right? And why did this happen to you? Recognize this kind of story? In this situation, the worst part is not knowing what to do. Let's investigate why you got tennis elbow.

Overuse

The most common cause of tennis elbow is overuse.[20] Lai et al (2018) noted that *"lateral epicondylitis is a significant source of pain and dysfunction resulting from repetitive gripping or wrist extension (lifting the hand up when your palm is facing down), radial deviation (turning the hand towards the thumb side), and/or forearm supination (palm up when the elbow is bent to 90 degrees)."*

When I start working with a new client, one of the first questions I ask them is, "How long have you been suffering?" Now regardless of how long they've actually had it (I do need to know this to effectively plan their treatment program) I want to know what changed three to six months **before** they started feeling their symptoms. Something changed.

Did you start a new workout regime? Did you start doing new exercises? Did you increase the weight on certain exercises? Sometimes it can be that. Did you start a new activity? Did you take up tennis? Did you renovate your house? Did you go traveling? Did you start a new job? Has your work set-up or your workstation changed? This can cause a change in stresses and strains around the elbows and can irritate tendons and other soft tissues. Have you spent time painting your garden fence? What have you been doing that flared this up? There's likely some kind of overuse in your history. The reason you need to find out what it was, is so that you can stop doing it, change it, or make it into a much kinder activity for your elbow. There are ways to change activities. It's not always about completely stopping something.

Stop and have a think right now:

When did my elbow pain start?

_____

_____

_____

What was the date 3 months before this?

_____

_____

_____

What was the date 6 months before this?

_____

_____

_____

What was I doing differently around those times?

_____

_____

_____

Hopefully, you may have uncovered what caused your elbow pain. If not, let's read on.

Altered biomechanics

The second cause can be altered or abnormal biomechanics. When you think about biomechanics, sports may jump to mind. You may think about tennis or golf. Think about different sports that you enjoy, and think about how you move as you're doing these activities.

But biomechanics is not always a sport-related thing. It could be the way you're painting your garden fence. You could be using an abnormal biomechanical movement to do that. Abnormal for you that is. Maybe you're awkwardly holding the brush. Maybe you have a problem with your shoulder that's having a knock-on effect on your elbow. Or maybe it could be overuse because you've been doing it for hours and hours on end, so you got tired and changed your technique. It can be as simple as that.

It could even be the way you're doing a particular activity at work. Descatha et al (2016) found *"an association between biomechanic exposure involving the wrist and/or elbow at work and the incidence of lateral epicondylitis."*

Direct trauma

The third cause can be a direct injury. Tennis elbow tends to be an overuse issue, but not always. You may have slipped, tripped, or bumped your elbow right on the tendon and created an inflammatory reaction that led to tennis elbow. A direct injury is a much less common cause of tennis elbow than overuse, but it can happen. Thankfully, the same strategies work to resolve it, regardless of the cause.

Compensation mechanism

The fourth cause can be a compensation mechanism for another injury. As I alluded to with the biomechanics, if you've hurt your shoulder, you use your arm differently and it's possible to irritate your elbow. Maybe you broke your wrist and you couldn't use that arm. Suddenly, the other arm is doing all the work and you irritate the tendon on that side. Indeed, a study done in the UK found a high correlation between tennis elbow in people who had a history of rotator cuff issues in their shoulder, carpal tunnel syndrome, or a De Quervains problem in the thumb.[21] Park et al (2021) found that *"female sex, dominant-side involvement, manual labor, and ipsilateral* (the same side) *rotator cuff tear were found to be risk factors for lateral epicondylitis."*

Antibiotics

One cause of tendon problems that most people don't know about is taking certain antibiotics.[22] Le Huec et al (1995) described *"epicondylitis after treatment with fluoroquinolone antibiotics."* But this is an unusual cause. If people suffer from tendon issues caused by taking antibiotics, it tends to lead to Achilles tendon problems, but other tendons can also be affected. I've worked with a handful of clients who developed tennis elbow in this way. So, sometimes it can be that if you're really searching for the cause. If I ask, "What happened?" and they respond with "I can't think of anything. Oh, wait, I had a chest infection and I had to take antibiotics for it." Maybe that was it.

Ergonomics

Poor ergonomics can be another contributing factor. Remember earlier when I mentioned workstation setup? Our bodies are designed to be in a nice upright, straight position. Think about your ear lobe, shoulder, and hips all being nicely aligned when you're standing or sitting. That's where our spine and bodies like to be.

However, most people adopt a "C" shaped curve in their spine when they're working on their computer, especially if they're working on a laptop. The "C" shaped curve puts a lot of pressure on your spine, especially your neck, as you have to crank it up to see the screen if your lower back is rounded. This can put pressure on the nerves that come out of the neck and go all the way down to the tips of your fingers. There is a big correlation between tendon problems and nerve irritation. If you irritate a nerve or pinch a nerve, that can cause a tendon to become inflamed.

The overuse of the keyboard, mouse, trackpad, and phone can also contribute to tendon irritation. Look for the strategies in chapter 6 to help with these specific issues.

Central sensitization

Central sensitization is a hypersensitivity of the nervous system that occurs when someone has suffered pain for three months or longer. Interestingly enough, this can then predispose you to further injuries, specifically tendon issues like tennis elbow. So, you may have suffered from sciatica for years and can't find any other specific reason that you developed tennis elbow. But your sciatica likely predisposed you to injuring your elbow, so it didn't take much to irritate it.

Treede et al (2015) stated *"The International Association for the Study of Pain defines chronic pain as persistent or recurrent pain lasting longer than 3 months."* Dahlhamer et al (2018) found "it *represents a major healthcare problem worldwide, affecting 20% of adults."* That's 1 in every 5 people suffering from chronic pain! Some research puts this number even higher at 1 in every 3 people!

Raffaeli et al (2021) stated *"chronic pain is not a mere temporal extension of acute pain, as it lacks the warning function of physiological nociception, and it is maintained by factors pathogenetically and physically remote from the initial cause, such as central sensitization."* Hmm, ok, hang on. What the heck does that all mean? Let's explore it.

Chronic pain is not a mere temporal (in your head) extension of acute (short term - less than 3 months) pain, as it lacks the warning function of physiological nociception (danger signals from your body caused by physical injury), and it is maintained by factors pathogenetically (the way you are made) and physically remote from the initial cause (not near the site of the injury), such as central sensitization.

Why does this even matter? Well, if the researchers have found that something is keeping your pain going, but it's not at the original site of the injury, doesn't it follow that just treating your elbow (the original site of the injury), might not give you the relief you are looking for? Let's peel back the layers a little further...

Jespersen et al (2013) *"assessed pain sensitivity and spreading hyperalgesia (an increased sensitivity to feeling pain and extreme response to pain) in lateral epicondylalgia and found that pressure-pain threshold and tolerance were on average reduced by over 30% in tennis elbow sufferers compared to non-sufferers when testing their forearms. But more interestingly, this was also the case when they tested their lower legs too."* Why would tennis elbow sufferers have reduced tolerance to pressure pain in their legs? This is surmised to be due to the varying duration of symptoms (the longer they had suffered, the more pain they experienced) and different degrees of central sensitization. In other words, the longer they had suffered, the more likely they were to feel pain AND it spread in their body.

Think of a pebble being dropped into a pond. The ripples travel further and further out as time goes on. Now think of your tennis elbow as the epicenter, where the pebble drops in. It's easy to see that the symptoms may travel as readily as the ripples.

Previtali et al (2022) found *"features of both central and peripheral sensitisation can be constantly detected in lateral epicondylalgia."* So we know this happens. Why is it so very rarely addressed by healthcare professionals? This goes back to the fact that the healthcare profession is a bit like a tendon - it's very, Very, VERY slow to change!

Yang et al (2019) defined chronic pain as *"a condition in which pain progresses from an acute to a chronic state and persists beyond the healing process. Chronic pain impairs function and decreases patients' quality of life."* They also described the structural and functional changes in brain structures that accompany the chronification of pain.

Yes, you read that right. Suffering pain for a prolonged time changes your brain. If the changes that chronic pain has made in your brain are not reversed, your body cannot fully heal. Your tendon will stay degenerated and you will not recover. This is why strategies to reverse these changes are crucial.

Thankfully the medical community has learned a lot about chronic pain over the past few years and there are simple strategies that you can start doing from today to help reverse the chronic pain changes in your brain. You'll find some of these listed in Chapter 7.

Although there are several reasons that people get tennis elbow, the strategies to heal it are all similar.

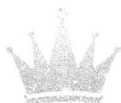

CHAPTER 4

The Most Common Mistakes You Can Make With Tennis Elbow

1. Doing nothing
2. Just treating the pain with pain pills
3. Having injections
4. Undergoing surgery
5. Relying on a brace, strap or clasp
6. Searching for the ONE thing that will fix your elbow
7. Over resting
8. Trusting exercises you found online
9. Not doing physical therapy (physio)
10. Hoping massage will cure it
11. Relying on passive electrotherapy treatments

1. Doing nothing

The biggest mistake has to be, doing nothing. Why suffer when you don't have to? Many people have issues that could be helped really simply and even completely resolved with the right treatment. So, why don't they do it?

Maybe someone didn't know what to do, so they did nothing. Simply said, the person suffering didn't know there was a way to solve their problem. Maybe their doctor had told them that it was "Just their age" and "They had to live with it" or to "Just take these pills". Maybe the surgeon had told them that surgery was the only option, but they didn't want to undergo such a drastic procedure, so accepted the fact that nothing could be done.

You might get to the point where you are so fed up with it hurting that you don't do anything. You don't play tennis. You don't play your musical instrument. You don't play with your kids. You don't lift your groceries. You don't do any of these things because you know it's going to hurt. That's not living.

Please remember that there is always something that can be done. There actually may be several little things that can be done, which when added together can build to big changes over time. I guarantee there will be strategies in this book that you won't have tried before. Have faith and trust the process. This has worked for thousands of people and can work for you, but **only if you do it.**

2. Just treating the pain with pain pills

Everyone in the healthcare professions are helpers. Go and see a doctor with a problem and they want to help. They look in their "toolbox" and match something that can help you with your symptoms. For example, if you have pain, they may offer you a painkiller. If you have muscle spasm, they may offer you a muscle relaxer medication. If you have inflammation, they may offer you an anti-inflammatory pill. These tools can help. Painkillers block the pain messages from getting through to your brain, where you would perceive it. But they don't heal the cause of the pain. Muscle relaxers can relax muscle spasm to allow you to feel much looser, until the medication wears off, and without healing the **cause** of the muscle spasm. Anti-inflammatory pills reduce inflammation because that's how they work to allow you to feel better. But they don't heal the cause of the inflammation.

These tools can be helpful during the healing process. For instance, if you are unable to sleep due to pain, medication can be helpful to allow you to get a good night's sleep. Sleep deprivation can be a form of torture, as any new parent would agree. We heal when we sleep. So, if you can't sleep you can't heal.

However, there can be side effects. Look at the side of any bottle of medication and you can read about the side effects. What are you potentially doing to your liver, your stomach, your body? Thankfully, there are other ways to achieve similar effects. You'll learn some strategies later in the book.

There is a difference between symptom resolution (relief of pain) and healing the tendon. Cook et al (2016) noted *"addressing pain is critical; however, interventions directed solely at pain have a minimal effect on the associated kinetic chain deficits or tissue capacity and may result in the recurrence of pain."*

This is exactly why it's imperative to heal the tendon. You'll learn about strategies for both "symptom resolution" AND true "tendon healing" as you navigate through the book.

3. Having injections

Cortisone steroid injections used to be the go-to treatment for tennis elbow. My own Mum had two. It is now known that cortisone steroids can do more harm than good in soft tissue problems like tennis elbow. Cortisone can cause soft tissues to degenerate. Buchanan et al (2022) reported *"rupture of the tendons with repeated steroid injections."* Coombes et al (2010) found *"evidence to suggest that beyond 26 weeks, patients who received a corticosteroid injection were more symptomatic than those who received no treatment or physical therapy".* The injected patients felt MORE symptoms than those who did not receive injections.

Platelet-rich plasma or PRP, is another type of injection that is popular among tennis elbow sufferers looking for relief. Not all PRP is created equally. Many doctors offer PRP and the strength and type of PRP depends on the kit they have. How do you know which is the best for your particular problem? The answer is, you don't. It can be a shot in the dark, so to speak (excuse the pun).

Karjalainen et al (2021) reviewed current evidence on the benefit and safety of autologous whole blood (AB) or platelet-rich plasma (PRP) injection for treatment of people with lateral elbow pain. Their review of 32 studies involving 2337 participants found:

"Data in this review do not support the use of autologous blood or PRP injection for treatment of lateral elbow pain. These injections probably provide little or no clinically important benefit for pain or function (moderate-certainty evidence), and it is uncertain (very low-certainty evidence) whether they improve treatment success and pain relief > 50%, or increase withdrawal due to adverse events. Although risk for harm may not be increased compared with placebo injection (low-certainty evidence), injection therapies cause pain and carry a

small risk of infection. **With no evidence of benefit, the costs and risks are not justified."**

O'Dowd (2022) concluded *"no long-term physiological benefits were reported to justify the invasive and costly technique of obtaining, producing, and implementing PRP."*

Simental-Mendia et al (2020) showed *"PRP injection was not superior to placebo (saline injection) for relieving pain and joint functionality in chronic lateral epicondylitis."*

Linnanmaki et al (2020) showed that *"PRP or autologous blood injections did not improve pain or function at 1 year of follow-up in people with lateral epicondylitis compared with those who were given a saline injection. They concluded that until or unless future randomized trials convincingly show a benefit either to PRP or autologous blood injections, they recommend against their use in patients with lateral epicondylitis."*

Stem cell injections are another avenue being explored for healing tennis elbow. This too is in the early stages of research. Therefore, the answer is we don't know if it works. The same can be said for enzyme injections, vitamin injections, indeed, any kind of injections. Have you ever wondered why insurance companies don't cover these newer treatment techniques? It's because their effectiveness hasn't been completely demonstrated. Cutts et al (2019) found that *"botox did not represent a definitive cure for this condition."* Yalcin et al (2022) investigated *"hyaluronic acid injections which showed no benefits whatsoever."*

Recently, I spoke with a client who had been in agony since a PRP injection 3 weeks prior. On chatting with him and trying to figure out exactly what was going on with him, it became apparent that the actual physical mechanism of the injection seemed to be the causative factor in his flare-up. It was irrelevant to the substance that had been injected. This anecdotal finding sits in line with research showing that patients who were suffering from tendon issues, who had multiple injections into the tendon, suffered for longer than those patients who didn't have injections and ultimately had a worse outcome.[6] As mentioned previously, injections are unnecessary in the treatment of resolving tennis elbow.

4. Undergoing surgery

Johns et al (2020) stated *"the available evidence supports the use of non-operative treatment modalities in managing this condition. When comparing the different operative treatments described, there appears to be no significant advantage of intervention over the natural history of lateral epicondylitis."* Basically, those patients who underwent surgery did not do any better than patients who did not.

But if you go and see a surgeon with a problem they are going to look in their toolbox to see if they can offer you a solution to your problem. The best surgeons I work with, are the ones who turn patients away. Let that sink in for a moment.

These are the surgeons that will say "Surgery is not the right option for you. There are better options for your solution, but I don't have them." These surgeons refer patients to other healthcare providers for more conservative treatment. They may also only spend a really short amount of time with you, they are not being rude, they just know that they don't have the solution your problem needs. In other words, you are not their patient because you don't need surgery.

Go and see enough different surgeons, however, and you will find someone who will perform surgery on you. They may suggest a "Try it and see" surgery. I advocate a "Try everything else first and even then, get a second opinion if you need to" approach. Your body will thank you for it, like my husband thanked me.

In 2013, my husband thought he had stomach flu, but it gradually got worse until he ended up in Urgent Care. It was six days before Christmas and my son's kindergarten class was performing their Holiday Show when I got a text from him, telling me that Urgent Care was referring him to the Emergency Room. I arranged for a friend to watch the kids and met him at the Emergency Room. The staff in the ER didn't know what was going on with my husband, so he was to be admitted for further investigations.

The following day my husband underwent a CT scan that came back inconclusive. He was steadily getting worse. They tried introducing a nasogastric tube, which is a tube that goes up your nose and down your esophagus into the stomach, to see if they could release the pressure building in his abdomen. It didn't work. He continued to decline.

Three days before Christmas he called me early in the morning to say he was going into surgery. I called the hospital to speak with the surgeon as I was driving to drop the kids off with my friend. The surgeon I spoke with told me they still couldn't figure out what was wrong with my husband, so they were taking him to surgery, to open him up from his breastbone to his pubic bone, to see what was going on in there. He would then be transferred to Intensive Care, after such a major surgery. I asked the surgeon to wait until I got to the hospital, and he told me that we would not be able to delay the surgery for long.

When I arrived at the hospital, I was greeted at the door by a nurse who had been a previous patient of mine, "What are you doing here?" she cried. I was so relieved to see a familiar face and I relayed the situation to her and told her that we needed a second opinion. She anxiously looked at me as she said "But they're all away skiing." Don't ever get sick around the holidays. But she told me she would search and find me someone. I couldn't thank her enough.

She called my husband's internal medicine physician to come and speak with me and this was pivotal. He came in to see us and I asked him "If this was your son, what would you do?" This question allows the doctor to see your situation in a different light. You can see the change in their eyes. The internist looked at me intently and he said "I would wait until tomorrow. You have 24 hours." I sighed a huge sigh of relief that we had some time. The surgeon that the nurse had found for our second opinion came in and agreed that surgery was necessary, but that my husband should wait until the following day.

The next day my husband had his surgery laparoscopically (keyhole). He didn't need to spend any time in Intensive Care and was able to come home by the New Year. What a difference a day makes. My point is that had I agreed to the solution the first surgeon had suggested, my husband would have had a vastly different experience. He would have been left with a 10-inch scar and been severely disabled for some time with a very lengthy recovery.

Now, I know that my husband's situation was an acute medical condition, which is quite different from a long-term chronic problem like tennis elbow, but the principle is the same, second opinions can be invaluable. Surgeons, doctors, and other healthcare professionals offer different options for the same problem. The challenge the patient has is knowing which option to choose. Getting more than one opinion can be a way to help. Also, trying all conservative options, before starting with invasive options, is generally the best way to proceed.

5. Relying on a brace, strap or clasp

There are so many different devices marketed to Tennis Elbow sufferers. New ones come out all the time. One client I know is still searching for the brace that's going to work for him and he's already got five in his closet. He has spent over $800 on just one. He's searching for the magic brace that's going to make his elbow better. But guess what? It is not there.

Braces or straps can take pressure off the tendon, but once you put something external on your arm, the muscles will switch off. This is a big issue for full healing. Let me explain. When your elbow started to hurt, you will have changed the way you do things to try to prevent the pain. By doing this, you will have stopped using your arm to a degree. Whenever we stop using a muscle, it starts to waste within hours.

One study found a decrease in protein synthesis after just 6 hours of immobilization.[14] Protein is the substance that muscles are made from and as you use your muscles, the protein is consistently replenished. If protein stops being made in the muscles, that's going to cause wasting pretty quickly. Another study showed that muscle fiber size had decreased by 17% in just 72 hours of immobilization.[15] That's muscle wasting. Another study showed that immobilizing the forearm for just 9 days caused a 32.5% decrease in strength.[16] Imagine how much strength could be lost after 9 weeks, 9 months, or 9 years. A similar study found that it took women longer to regain their strength than their male counterparts.[17] These studies were done on healthy, uninjured individuals who had casts placed on their wrists for the research.

So, if you use a brace or strap, the muscles of the forearm will waste. Muscle weakness is one of the issues of tennis elbow. Phase 3 of the program is strengthening, which is essential as this is when you actually heal the tendon. However relying on a brace or strap will accentuate the weakness and therefore, slow the healing.

My advice is not to use a brace or a strap if you can help it. There may be times when you need one, such as moving to a new house, which was mentioned previously as something that can lead to flare-ups in tennis elbow, or you may be in a job where you have to use your arms and can't rest. One client was a sushi chef and just couldn't change the way he worked and couldn't slow down either. A strap was invaluable to allow him to continue his work. A recent study showed that sufferers who wore a wrist brace benefited from some pain relief.[37] Just don't become reliant on a strap or brace. The ultimate goal is to wean off and get back to doing all the things you want to do with no restrictions.

6. Searching for the one thing that will fix your elbow

Stasinopoulos (2016) stated *"the effectiveness of an exercise programme is low when it is applied as monotherapy."* In other words, it's more effective when combined with other things.

Reuter (2023) found *"a multimodal treatment approach that focuses on progressive exercise therapy is recommended."* There is no one thing. Tennis elbow is a multi-faceted condition and requires a combination of strategies to heal it. I brought together the most effective combination of these treatments into this program.

7. Resting too much

If someone sees you struggling with something, what do they say? "Take it easy." If someone sees you in pain, what do they say? "Rest it." These are the right things to do, but only for the first 3 days after an injury. After that point, the tissues start to heal and need normal stresses and strains going through them to heal strongly and efficiently.

But how do you know that it's safe to move? A Licensed Physical Therapist is a movement and injury specialist who has the knowledge and expertise needed to guide you through the healing process. The longer you defer getting back to doing your normal activities, the more the muscles will weaken. The more the muscles weaken, the harder it is to get back to doing all the things you love.

There are so many options to try, but which are the right ones for you? That's the challenge right there. How would you know which options are safe and effective for you to try? There are some helpful tips that you can start from today, that are safe for all. I'll walk you through these from chapter 6.

8. Trusting exercises you found online

Clients have told me, "Well, I tried these exercises on YouTube," because that's what everybody does. They go to Dr. Google, type in their diagnosis and learn about it. Or they go to YouTube and do the exercises, but depending on what's causing the issue, you might find the wrong exercises. The wrong exercises are going to make you worse.

The internet has a lot of answers, but you need to ensure that the answers you find are the answers to the questions you are asking. Better said, you need to know what you are searching for before plugging something like "Exercises for Tennis Elbow" into the search bar of YouTube. Wondering why? Go on. Try it. Right now. Let's see what comes up.

You back? Well... what did you find? A ton of exercises for tennis elbow, right? Yes, there's certainly a lot of advice out there. However, how do you know which are the right exercises to heal your elbow? You don't know. I can tell you that there is some great advice out there and there's also some terrible advice that will make you worse. So, what should you do? If you're like most people, you probably get completely overwhelmed by the amount of differing advice and so do nothing. Understandably so. You don't want to try something that might make it worse, and so it feels safer to stick with the status quo.

What if you're one of the people who found one of the videos that had a lot of views and some good comments under it? Narrowing it down like that makes sense. So, you try what they suggest, and it makes it hurt like heck. What do you do now? Is it supposed to feel like that? Who can you ask? Silence. So, you stop doing the new exercise and stick with what you know, which is sensible.

You can find videos that say "This 5 minute exercise for tennis elbow will cure you". Unfortunately, that's highly unlikely. If it was that simple, your doctor would have told you about it at your first appointment. What other symptoms have you got? What structures are involved? Is that exercise going to get you better? No, probably not because they're likely not the right exercise.

Can you get the exercises you need from YouTube? No. This assumes that tennis elbow is a simple condition that needs a simple solution to resolve it. This is not the case. Tennis elbow is a multi-faceted condition that can affect many different structures. However, the multi-faceted nature of this condition requires a much higher level of understanding to fully heal it so that it never comes back. If you don't address every aspect of your tennis elbow, you will not resolve it completely and it will return.

9. Not doing physical therapy (physio)

Kim et al (2021) showed *"patients who received physical therapy reported statistically and clinically improved scores in pain and function compared to placebo."* So doing physical therapy is helpful. Buchanan et al (2022) stated that *"patients who fail to follow through on their therapy plan frequently have a recurrence of symptoms."* But you actually have to do it!

10. Hoping massage will cure it

Is massage going to help? Yes, generally it is. Is massage going to cure tennis elbow? No, it isn't. Not by itself. Do you need to go and see a massage therapist? Only if you want to, but you don't have to as you can do the soft tissue treatment techniques that you need at home. You don't need somebody else to do that for you. Your elbow is a very accessible part of your body. You can get to it yourself. I'll teach you what you need to do in chapter 8.

11. Relying on passive electrotherapy treatments

Ultrasound does have a place with certain conditions and at certain times within those conditions. But ultrasound does not help tennis elbow. It's the same for any passive electrotherapy treatments like laser, interferential or EStim. None of these electrical modalities heal tennis elbow.[18]

What about extracorporeal shock wave therapy (ESWT)? I have never actually experienced this but have heard from people who have tried it that it's pretty painful. There has been lots of buzz about it healing tennis elbow – you may even have heard this yourself. Unfortunately, the research shows that it is not beneficial in the treatment of tennis elbow.[19]

Yoon et al (2020) found that *"extracorporeal shock wave therapy did not show clinically important improvement in pain reduction and grip strength in patients with lateral epicondylitis."* Cutts et al (2019) found it *"did not represent a definitive cure for this condition."* Indeed, Bargeri et al (2023) found *"patients undergoing extracorporeal shock wave therapy were reporting mild adverse events."*

Cheema et al (2022) noted *"the available evidence does not support the use of passive electrophysiotherapy modalities, TENS or ESWT in the treatment of lateral epicondylitis."*

However, it must be noted that TENS – which we know doesn't HEAL tennis elbow, and the previous study showed no benefit of TENS at 12 months, BUT, TENS is a treatment modality that can reduce pain, so may be helpful as in the early stage. This is the difference between symptom resolution and healing. If a client needs pain relief, it's perfectly acceptable to use TENS (or whatever feels good to them - as long as it causes no harm) for a short time to help with this. Most people are fully aware that TENS alone will not heal the tendon, but are using it to decrease symptoms to allow them to be able to do the other strategies that will take them towards healing.

Infrared is a form of heat. You may have heard about infrared saunas or lamps and the benefits that they have. However, you can get great benefits from a hot water bottle, a heating pad, a hot towel, or a hot shower. Please do not feel you have to spend money because you think that's the one thing that's going to make you better. It's not. You can get some great relief from things you already have around the house.

Keep reading to learn which strategies to start with and how to apply them.

TENNIS ELBOW QUEEN

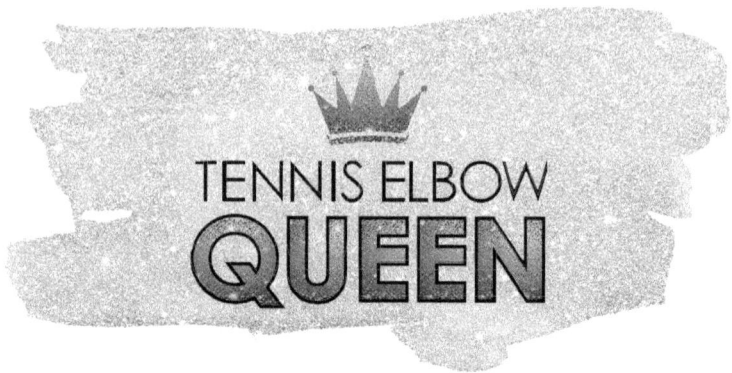

"After just a week my elbow is not hurting sharply like it was. I love the stretches and am now able to sleep comfortably through the night."

LR 34

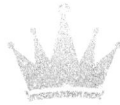

CHAPTER 5

The Comprehensive Program That Is Proven To Resolve Tennis Elbow

Now we get to the real crux: how to resolve tennis elbow. Here's what we'll be covering:

Phase 1 – Reducing symptoms

- Reduce symptoms
- Begin to calm the nervous system
- Start activity-specific visualization

Phase 2 - Normalizing soft tissues

- Normalize the soft tissues
- Regain range of motion
- Continue to calm the nervous system
- Add non-irritating activity-specific movements

Phase 3 – Strengthening

- Strengthening – core, neck, scapula, rotator cuff, and the forearm
- Forearm strengthening starts once the muscle tension of the forearm has normalized
- Activity-specific movements intensify

Phase 4 – Regaining endurance and function

- Regain endurance and function
- Return to high-intensity activities
- Return to sport - no restrictions
- Begin return to high-intensity activities once you have been completely pain-free for a week
- Specific nerve mobilizations (if they are needed)

These 4 phases make up the program and you'll learn about each phase in detail.

Some people ask, "Will tennis elbow just get better by itself?" Lai et al (2018) found that *"although most cases are self-limiting over several years, controversy exists regarding the best treatment strategy for chronic lateral epicondylitis."*

Let's unpack that a little. Self-limiting over several years! Do you want to be limited for several years? Nope. Didn't think so! And they specifically described **chronic** lateral epicondylitis. Chronic is defined as being present for 3 months or longer. So, they are basically saying that if you've had tennis elbow for 3 months or longer, it's going to limit you for several years before you feel better!

It doesn't have to be this way. I've seen patients who have suffered for:

- 17 months and were back playing tennis in 10 weeks.
- 18 months. That's Buddy, whose story you can read in the foreword to this book.
- 3 years, and became pain-free after just one session. (Now, this is not typical, but it can happen!)
- 5 years and this lady became pain-free in 3 weeks
- 7 years; this gentleman was back working out in the gym within four months
- Up to 30 years! Sufferers who have joined my free Facebook group – if you're not a member, you can join here:

https://www.facebook.com/groups/tenniselbowrelief

This is NOT OK. These people have been severely let down by the healthcare profession. But don't worry! You have the solution to avoiding this fate in your hands right now! Most of the sufferers who follow my program feel better in a matter of weeks and many are back playing tennis or golf within 3 months, NOT limited for several years.

The previous chapter contains everything I found when I first started working with Buddy. I trawled the research and found a whole lot of things that DON'T heal tennis elbow, but struggled to find much that did. So, I took my sports background knowledge of healing Achilles tendons quickly and efficiently, and applied it to Buddy's elbow. After a few months of trial and error and digging deep into his symptoms, we got the breakthrough that he wrote about in the foreword to this book. Since then, the program has changed and evolved in response to new research that emerges. I update my approach accordingly as new strategies and treatments come to light, and everything contained in this program is evidence-based. That means there is scientific research to support it and explain how and why it works.

The difference between symptom resolution and healing

There is a BIG difference between symptom resolution and actually healing the tendon. Some treatments and strategies can provide pain relief. If you were injected in the elbow with a local anesthetic, that would for sure deliver pain relief to you. However, it would NOT heal the tendon. Many of the "old school" treatments that were used for tennis elbow fit into this category. You may feel some relief from symptoms, but they are not healing the tendon. From time to time, someone joins my Facebook group who has had great success with a topical ointment and balm. Everyone clamors to find out about the "miracle cure". However, none of these topical treatments, or even any ONE strategy can heal the tendon.

Heales et al (2016) stated, *"Features of neuromuscular control differ between individuals with lateral epicondylalgia and pain-free controls. This implies potential central nervous system involvement and indicates that rehabilitation may be enhanced by consideration of neuromuscular control in addition to other treatments"*. This element of central sensitization has become the foundation of my program, and if it's not addressed, is the biggest reason that people "fail" therapy.

"Emma, can't I get all the information off the internet?" Well, yes and no. Most of the information that I gathered over the past 15 years, whilst I was working with my clients and collating it into the program that I now deliver, is all out there, but you've got to know where to look and, more importantly, you've got to know how to apply it. You've got to know what's good information and what's not. You've also got to know about the phases of healing. You're more than likely going to need to start with phase one, but what does that mean and why does it matter? Let me explain about the four phases of healing your elbow.

Over the years of helping people heal, I realized that the strategies I'd found to resolve tennis elbow, sat pretty neatly into 4 phases of healing. Additionally, this concept was described by Keijsers et al (2019) when they found that *"the different stages of tennis elbow need a different approach."*

Phase 1

Phase one is when you are feeling the symptoms. It's uncomfortable, and maybe you can't sleep at night. You can't do the activities you love or even simple day-to-day things. You can't pick up a cup of coffee or a bottle of water without feeling pain. Phase one treatment strategies start to settle down the symptoms. It resolves the sharp discomfort. It begins to relax the muscle tension. It helps you to start to feel a bit more normal. Once you've got yourself into a routine with phase one, you can move onto phase two.

Phase 2

Phase two normalizes the soft tissues and regains any range of motion you may have lost. Now that is not necessarily the range of motion in your elbow. It may be the range of motion in your neck or your shoulder or shoulder blade, depending on how things are moving. It's about addressing tissue tightness;

forearm tightness, and upper trapezius (shoulder stress muscles) tightness. Getting things moving normally helps things feel much more normal. There's quite an overlap from phase one to phase two and together they can start helping quickly.

Phase 3

Phase three is my favorite phase, it's all about strengthening. You will have weakened muscles if you have been suffering with tennis elbow. The reason for this is that it hurts, so you don't use your arm as much as you would normally. As soon as you stop using the muscles, they start to weaken. You need to strengthen everything back up. There are different ways of strengthening. There is a way that will irritate you and there's a way that will heal you. The magic happens when you know which is which.

Phase 4

Phase four is going to be your favorite as you'll get back to doing everything you want to do. It'll get you back to playing tennis, playing golf, running, biking, cycling, rowing, working out, playing the drums, playing the guitar, playing the violin or the viola, swimming, picking your kids up, picking up the groceries, renovating your house, using a screwdriver, all of those things that you can't do right now; even picking up that glass of water, or cup of coffee. It gets you back to doing everything you want to do with no restrictions.

How do you know what you need to do for each of the phases? The information is all out there. Will you find it packaged neatly, so you can understand it? Probably not. If you've ever read a research article, particularly a medical research article, they're pretty dry (there are many listed at the end of this book). There are not many pictures and they're quite repetitive. The outcome of all of them is that more research is needed because it always is. We are always learning. That's why the program evolves. I change things as new research comes out.

This program is successful. It's really successful. The most memorable clients are the people who have tried everything before; they've got the brace, they've done ice, they've been to PT and they end up sitting in front of a surgeon and saying, "I want surgery". This is exactly what happened to my very first tennis elbow client. You read his story in the foreword to this book.

The very first client that I helped came to me by default. Let's go back to 2008. I was working at my local hospital as a physical therapist in outpatients, seeing everybody, backs, necks, shoulders, knees, a little bit of everything. By chance, I shared an office with an occupational therapist and another physical therapist. At the end of every day, we would write our notes together.

One day the occupational therapist was writing her notes and she put her notes down, sat back in her chair, looked at me, and said, "I've got this patient". You always know that you're going to get a story when somebody says that. So, I put my pen down and I sat back to listen. She told me about her client. He'd searched for help everywhere in California. He had seen everyone around Los Angeles. He was a professional drummer, and he couldn't drum because he had tennis elbow. So, he ended up sitting in front of a surgeon and he said to her, "I've been everywhere. I've tried everything. I'm a professional drummer and I can't drum. Give me surgery on this elbow so I can drum."

This is why I love the surgeon I work with. She said, "No, I don't know exactly what treatment you've tried up to now, so I want you to go and see my therapists at the hospital first." He was upset as he said, "I want surgery, I need this fixed now." She said, "I'm not going to do anything until you go see them. I don't know who you've seen and what they've done. You need to go and see my people first. Then, if you still have problems, come back to see me." He wasn't happy at having to wait longer, but he did set up the appointment with the occupational therapist, who the surgeon wanted him to see.

So, my friend, the occupational therapist, had treated him for a few sessions for his elbow. He was asking all kinds of different questions. For example, he was saying to her, "Do you think my thoracic spine can affect my elbow? I read somewhere that if you treat the thoracic spine, it can help tennis elbow." The thoracic spine is the mid back. My occupational therapist friend is a Certified Hand Therapist. She is one of the most knowledgeable, experienced, amazing therapists I've ever worked with. She deals with clients who have shoulder, elbow, wrist, and hand problems. She doesn't deal with the thoracic spine. So, this was her question to me. She said, "I have this patient who's tried all these things. He's asked me about treatment for his thoracic spine. What do you think?" I knew that for sure, the cervical spine (the neck) could affect the elbow, but I wasn't sure about the thoracic spine. So, I said, "Put him on my list. Let me see him."

So, we met, and I think he probably rolled his eyes again; somebody else, yet another pair of eyes looking at him. I worked with him over a period of months and we peeled back the layers of what needed addressing. He was right. He did need work on his thoracic spine, as well as his neck, his shoulder blade, his shoulder, his upper trapezius muscle, his elbow, wrist, and hand, plus the nerves that go down his arm. He needed everything. So, we went through and addressed everything.

This included coming up with a new way of treating tennis elbow, to ensure that it fully healed once and for all. He would do the exercises himself at home and integrate the other strategies that I had added to address all the different elements of his issue. Within 6 months, he was able to get back to playing the drums. All these years later, he's still doing great. His tennis elbow is completely resolved. He continues to play drums, he writes music, he is successful, and he is pain-free. Did he need surgery? No. Did he need injections? No. So, I tell you this story to know that there is hope when you find the right person who has the solution to the problem that you have.

Recap

To recap, addressing chronic pain and central sensitization is crucial and is why you will start working on calming your nervous system from day 1. Is this a one-and-done solution? No. We've established that no "one" thing will heal your tendon, but a combination of factors will. How long will you need to do these things to see a difference? Most clients see a positive change in weeks, not months. Some even in a few days. However, Palmer et al (2023) showed that *"exercise interventions that were 12 weeks or longer altered brain function and improved pain and/or quality of life outcomes."* So plan on following everything in this plan for at least 3 months. Let's begin your journey.

TENNIS ELBOW QUEEN

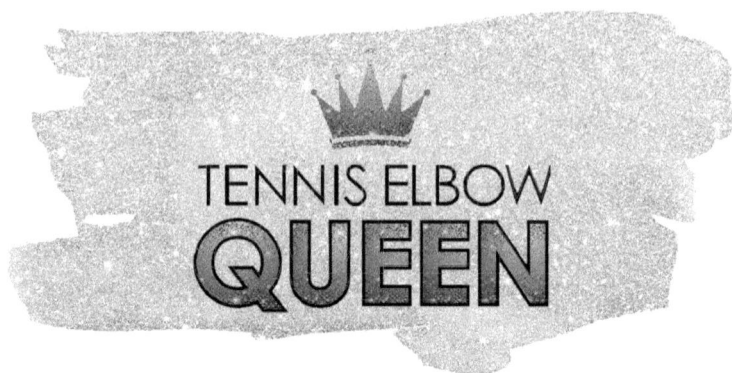

66 It's great to not feel pain in my elbow again now after such a long time. I had first felt my elbow in Summer. By September, I went to PT which didn't work. Then I tried acupuncture which didn't help. My orthopedic doctor suggested a cortisone shot; it felt better for three weeks, then recurred. Another ortho suggested PRP which I did, but it didn't help. I had an MRI and the elbow specialist said I had to rest for 3 months. But I still had pain. Then someone told me about Emma. I was very skeptical initially, but within 6 weeks I was pain free and hitting golf balls. Thank you Emma. 99

AA 62

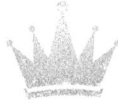

CHAPTER 6

Phase 1
Reducing Symptoms

This section contains the self-help strategies that everyone suffering from tennis elbow needs regardless of how long they have suffered. However, if you've suffered for 3 months or longer, you will also need the nervous system related strategies in chapter 7. Every single strategy can be started today, right now at home with minimal equipment. There's a lot that you can do to help and we're going to go through each action item in detail.

Phase 1 Goals
- Reduce symptoms
- Start activity-specific visualization if applicable

Phase 1 Strategies

1. Relative rest
2. Heat
3. Ice
4. Posture
5. Ergonomics
6. Braces
7. Tape
8. Sleep
9. Pills
10. Topicals
11. Nutrition
12. Nutritional supplements
13. Hydration
14. Cardio
15. Progressive relaxation
16. Visualization

Now, I know this seems like a long list and you're probably already thinking you can't fit all of that into your day. But, don't worry, you might not need all of them and it's not forever, it's just for now. That is one of my catchphrases, and it's true. Think about Phase 1 as setting the foundation for the rest of your healing journey. If you don't have a solid foundation, anything that comes later is on shaky ground and cannot be as effective.

Many of these items take just 5 minutes per day. Some strategies will help you get to the next stage, and others I hope you will do for as long as you can. Every element in this program has been proven to optimize healing, allowing you to heal in the fastest and most effective way possible.

1.   Relative rest

Keep yourself as comfortable as possible.

Bhabra et al (2016) stated that *"the primary aim of "relative rest" is to halt the injury process by removing mechanical overload, providing the tendon a chance to repair itself through the restriction and modification of provocative daily activities."* I couldn't have put it better myself.

But what does this mean for you? Relative rest means avoiding anything that makes your injury hurt. You're not taking to your bed or putting your arm in a sling, but you do need to avoid things that irritate it. Sometimes, this is easier said than done if the irritating factor is your job or your sport. However, there may be things in your day that you don't actually have to do. You might want to do them but ask yourself if you really have to do them.

For example, a client who irritated her elbow by cleaning her baseboards. When I asked her why she was doing this irritating activity, she replied that they were dirty and needed cleaning before her family came over for a holiday dinner. This is not an essential activity. She wanted her baseboards to be clean, but they really didn't need to be done. I'll bet her family didn't even notice her baseboards, but they sure noticed her wincing in pain when she reached for her wine glass. Get the point? There are certain activities that we can choose to do, or not.

2.   Heat the heck out of it

Heat for 10 minutes every hour through the day.

Heat is your friend! One of my favorite phrases is "Heat the heck out of it!". You can check out my helpful product list to see the heat pads many clients love. Heat is INCREDIBLY helpful!

The theory behind heat application is that it:

- Increases circulation - great for a tissue with a poor blood supply and therefore challenged with healing.

- Decreases muscle tension - which takes force off the tendon allowing it to heal.

- *"Increased muscle fiber conduction velocity and improved binding of contractile proteins (actin, myosin)"* (Chaabene et al, 2019). Basically, the muscle can work better.

- Feels way nicer than ice - use heating as a little bit of "you" time, along with knowing that you are healing your tendon in the fastest way possible.

"But Emma, I thought I was supposed to put ice on my elbow." Heat your forearm and elbow unless it is acute (very recent), or if you feel you've irritated your elbow, then, you will ice your elbow instead. If you have any acute injury, you need three days of ice. But you can still heat your neck, shoulder, and forearm. It's helpful to get heat into the tissues to relax the muscles. This is why it's often the first thing I recommend.

You're going to need a heating pad, a hot towel, or a hot water bottle. You may stand slightly longer under a hot shower because it feels good. Heat from any source can work. However, heating pads tend to be easier to use throughout the day. There's also a recommended equipment list in the book bonuses:

http://bit.ly/TE-bookbonuses

You don't have to go and stand under the shower all the time. It can be nice when you shower, but heat must be done frequently throughout the day. I used to recommend heat 2-3 times a day, but a couple of clients healed faster and better by using heat more frequently. So ideally, heat for 10 minutes every hour. The forearm is often very tight because the body recognizes an injury to the tendon and wants to take the stress and strain away from that tissue. That stress and strain will go elsewhere and can make the muscles tight. If the muscles stay tight, the tendon will struggle to heal. So, relaxing the muscles with heat helps.

The heating pads I particularly like are the ones that you heat in the microwave. They tend to mold around the area a little better than electric ones, which don't tend to be as malleable. The microwave ones also have a bit of weight as they have beads, seeds, or corn inside, and the gentle pressure on the muscles can also help with relaxation. If you already have a heating pad or a hot water bottle, go and get it right now and come back. Go on, go and do it. Right now. It's going to help.

Make sure that you are comfortable when you heat. If you're not, change it. You don't want to damage your skin. If you use heat that is too hot for you it's possible to cause skin to discolor. I don't just mean the normal redness that occurs with heat application. It's a more permanent discoloration that does not fade after a few minutes like redness would. It stays for a few weeks and indicates damage to the skin. When you put heat on, you want to feel a comfortable warmth, that feels relaxing. If it gets too hot your muscles will tense up. That is not what you're trying to achieve. You are trying to get relaxation of the tissues, not tightening them up. Tension can pull on the tendon and make it hurt. The relaxation will relieve tension in the muscle and, therefore, on the tendon and so allow it to start healing.

3. Ice, Ice, Baby

Ice for 3 days if you've irritated it.

Radecka et al (2022) found *"one application of local cryotherapy (ice) reduces the pain and increases pain-free grip and muscle excitation, and seems to delay muscle fatigue."* Therefore, it can be a useful strategy in the early stages for getting pain under control.

Manias et al (2006) found *"an exercise programme consisting of eccentric and static stretching exercises (which you'll learn in phases 2 and 3) had reduced the pain in patients with lateral elbow tendinopathy at the end of the treatment and at the follow-up whether or not ice was included."* So, for this reason, the application of ice is NOT routinely needed. However, you can use ice for comfort should it feel good to you. Ice can be useful at numbing pain, allowing you to do the other things you need to do for healing. For example, some people find using ice before bed helpful in getting a better night's sleep.

If you have irritated your elbow with an activity like moving house, which caused your elbow to flare up, ice can be helpful during the following 3 days to reduce any acute inflammation that may have been stirred up by the unaccustomed activity. After this time, you can switch back to heat.

The tendon does not have a good blood supply, so you want to increase the blood supply to the tendon as much as you can and heat can do that beautifully. If you think about when you take a heating pad off, the skin is pink underneath. You've got your circulation going. The same can be said for ice. If you put an ice pack on your elbow and leave it on for 5 to 10 minutes before you take it off, the skin is going to be pink underneath. You've got the circulation going, but ice then constricts the blood vessels. You're not going to get quite the same effect as with the heat, which is why we use heat and ice for different reasons.

Use ice to help with swelling because it constricts the vessels. Heat opens everything up, and you get a big influx of blood into the area. That's the reason you don't use heat in the acute phase because you don't want a big rush of blood to an area that is very recently injured. It's already bleeding. If you put heat on and get extra blood flow into the area it will make it worse. Therefore, for the first three days of any new injury, ice only. After the first three days, you can choose. Most people prefer heat. Every now and again, somebody will prefer ice. That's okay. It's a personal choice, but just know that heat will get the blood flow going better than ice. However, if ice is helpful for you to numb the pain, use it.

You do not need a big ice pack for this. A little ice pack right on the irritated area can be immensely helpful. A packet of frozen peas can work. Just don't eat the peas afterward because when they've been on your elbow, they will thaw and then you're going to refreeze them. Put a small packet of frozen peas into a Ziploc bag, just in case it splits, and you can use that on your elbow.

When you're using ice, you need to make sure you protect your skin. You've got your ice pack out of the freezer and to protect the skin you can wrap a damp tea towel around it before you put it on your elbow. You do not want the ice pack sticking to your skin because when you take it off, your skin can become damaged. You can rip the top layer of skin off and then you won't be able to ice or heat it until it has healed. Don't slow your healing down. To be doubly sure it's not going to stick, use a very thin layer of oil on your skin. It can be any kind of oil. It doesn't have to be anything special. You can use vegetable oil or olive oil from your kitchen. If you want to use vitamin E oil, that's entirely up to you, but you do not need anything special. Just use a thin layer of oil, wrap it with a damp towel, and get ice on for 10 minutes maximum. If it becomes uncomfortable, take it off. Any strategy you use needs to be completely pain-free. If it's not, something's wrong.

4. Posture rules

Good posture reduces abnormal stress and strain on the tissues.

Keijsers et al (2019) found *"occupational factors that contribute to the onset of tennis elbow are characterized by strenuous manual activities for the wrist and/or elbow which consist of both force and posture."* That is, the position you spend your time in. If you did nothing else, but improve your posture, you would feel so much better. We spend so much time and energy trying to figure out which exercise to do, which supplement to take, or which doctor is the best one to see, when in fact, if you just sat a little straighter and kept your spine in neutral, maybe you wouldn't have to focus so much on the other things.

Sitting puts a lot of stress and strain on the spine, neck, nerves and other soft tissues. Tendons and nerves are very closely correlated. If you have a tendon problem such as tennis elbow, you are 86% likely to have some kind of nerve issue too.[27]

The spine is designed to be curvy. The little curve in the lower back is called the lumbar lordosis.

Sitting in poor posture is going to make the healing process longer. This is because when the lower back is in a poor C-shaped position, you have to lift your head up to see in front of you. This

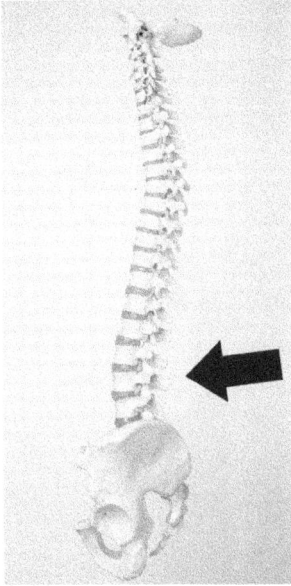

can lead to the soft tissues around your neck, including nerves, being irritated.

Being in a good posture with your earlobe, shoulder, and hips in a nice straight line (if you're looking from the side), is going to help to optimize your healing time by taking the abnormal stress and strain off the tissues.

To achieve the optimal position when you are sitting, move your hips to the back of the chair and use the backrest, making sure you've got something supporting your lumbar lordosis, the little curve in your lower back. If you have a chair that has a lumbar support, use it by just resting back against it. If your chair doesn't have a

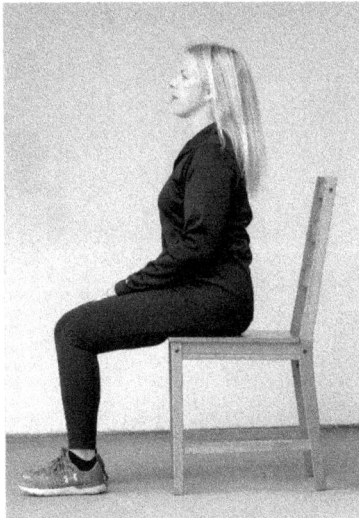

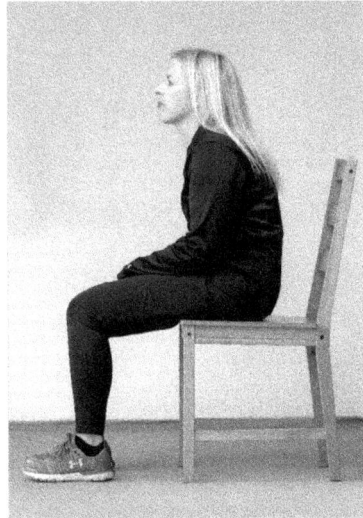

lumbar support, you can roll up a towel and use it in that space. If you are out, you can roll up your sweater or jacket and use it as a support.

You've probably got a lumbar support in your car that you can tweak to fit you and be more comfortable. If it's there, use it. It may be similar in your office chair. Sitting in good posture, and having your lumbar lordosis supported, is where the spine is designed to be. It's where there's the least amount of abnormal stress and strain going through it.

If you have an irritated nerve associated with your tennis elbow, you may feel the nerve symptoms more when you are sitting at your desk. If you get a tingling, pins and needles or a numbness sensation, you will likely move and it will resolve. However, if you go back to sitting in the same position, it's going to keep coming back.

Your challenge for today is to sit in better posture. Set the timer on your phone for 20 minutes, when the timer goes off, stand up, sit back down in good posture, and reset your timer. What happens when you are sitting and working on your laptop, watching TV, or surfing the internet, you will get sucked into that activity, and before you know it, all your good intentions will be gone. That's the reason for setting your timer for 20 minutes because, after 20 minutes, you're probably in the C-shaped curve. You need a reminder. If you don't have an external reminder like your phone timer, you may get an internal reminder, which will be pain.

This strategy does not take you away from your desk or your work. It just breaks up the day. This can be transformational. I have known several clients who have started with this one strategy and it makes such a difference to how they're feeling. You stand up and sit down. It's less than a second. But if you do it consistently throughout the day, you will notice a difference.

"Can I just wear one of those devices that hold me in a good posture?" The answer is yes, you could, but when you put something external on, it may pull and force you into a good position. But the tissues underneath, the muscles, will switch off. As a result, if you wear a back support or one of the posture devices that go around your shoulders and pull your shoulders back to try and keep you upright, that will cause a weakening of the postural muscles and you may become completely reliant on that device.

Our spine is designed to have curves. These curves allow our spine to move in the way that it is designed to and also to absorb stress and strain most effectively. If those curves flatten out, the spine is less effective at absorbing strain and tissues may become damaged. This is where the term "neutral spine" comes in. Neutral spine means the naturally occurring position where there is the least amount of abnormal stress or strain on the spine.

Let's find your neutral spine position right now. Focus on the position that you are currently in. How does your spine feel? Is it comfortable? If not, why not?

Arch your back as much as you can comfortably, then round it in the opposite direction as much as you comfortably can. Go from one extreme of the movement to the other extreme of the movement a few times. Make a mental note of how it feels when you are at the end of each motion. Now stop yourself in the middle. Feel how there's less stress and strain on your spine now? Welcome to neutral.

5. Ergonomics

Use your chair and wrist rests correctly.

Remember this piece of research from the previous section? Keijsers et al (2019) found *"occupational factors that contribute to the onset of TE are characterized by strenuous manual activities for the wrist and/or elbow which consist of both force and posture."* Well, this also applies to ergonomics.

Many people ask, "What's the best office chair or the best mouse?" and the answer is "It depends." We're all different, and what's right for one person isn't necessarily going to be right for another. The best advice I can give is "try them out".

You need a supportive chair, ideally with a high backrest that extends up to allow your head to rest on it. Think of the supportive seat with a headrest in your car. A lumbar support is very helpful but can be added as an external cushion. Your feet should rest comfortably on the floor. If you're a little on the short side, like me, using a footrest is essential to stop you from dangling. Make sure you are nice and upright. Scoot your chair underneath the desk so that you are in a nice straight position. In addition, make sure that the monitor is at eye level.

If you work on a laptop, you have to look down. If you are going to sit for eight hours a day working on a laptop, that's going to be a problem for your tissues. Raise the laptop up and use it as the monitor. Have a separate keyboard and mouse down below, and then you can work on a laptop perfectly well in a beautiful posture. It is essential to use wrist rests for both the keyboard and the mouse. You can see the ones I use in the equipment list.

Standing desks give you the option to change your position and avoid the poor position of sitting all day. It's important to be able to vary the position, as most people are not comfortable standing for prolonged periods either.

6. Biomechanics

Have an experienced coach analyze your movements.

Brukner et al (2012) stated that *"tennis players can benefit from additional sport-specific advice. Technique errors that are considered to predispose to the etiology of tennis elbow are (1) a faulty backhand technique with the elbow leading, (2) excessive forearm pronation during a forehand topspin, and (3) excessive wrist flexion during a service."* Additional potential risk factors are racket type, grip size, string tension, court surface and weight of the ball. These factors affect biomechanical loading of the elbow during tennis.

These issues and more can be alleviated by a knowledgeable tennis coach. If you'd like a recommendation in your area, reach out to me at Emma@TennisElbowQueen.com and I'll connect you with a great coach.

7. Braces

Use a wrist extension brace for the first 2 weeks and then a forearm strap up to 12 weeks only.

Shahabi et al (2020) found *"physiotherapy interventions compared to counterforce braces (forearm strap) have better effects, especially over the long term. However, counterforce braces may have better effects on pain in younger people (<45 years old) over the short term (<6 weeks)."*

Altan (2008) showed that *"a wrist extension splint was effective at decreasing pain in the first 2 weeks and either the wrist* *extension splint or a counterforce strap were effective in the early stages. **Clinical relevance:** The results suggest that counterforce bracing is a reasonable strategy to alleviate pain over the short term. However, the subgroup analysis suggests that factors such as age may have a role in their effectiveness."*

Bisset et al (2014) found *"counterforce braces had an immediate positive effect in participants with lateral epicondylalgia, without differences between interventions and similar to a no-brace control condition. Therefore, while the use of a brace may help manage immediate symptoms related to lateral epicondylalgia, the choice of which brace to use may be more a function of patient preference, comfort, and cost."*

Kroslak et al (2019) found *"the counterforce brace provides a significant reduction in the frequency and severity of pain in the short term (2-12 weeks), as well as overall elbow function at 26 weeks, compared with the placebo brace."*

Although, Barati et al (2019) showed *"minimal differences between improvements made with a forearm strap and an elbow sleeve."*

Heales et al (2020) Found *"evidence shows that forearm orthoses can immediately reduce pain during contraction and improve pain-free grip strength in individuals with lateral elbow tendinopathy. However, a static wrist orthosis did not improve pain-free grip strength."*

Now, that being said, you don't need to rush out and buy fancy braces. There are all kinds of braces available for tennis elbow. The classic one is the strap that goes around your forearm. Most people don't know how to use those correctly and they put them right over the area that hurts. It's supposed to go underneath the sore spot, on the muscles, and it goes on as tightly as you can have it without your hand going blue or tingling. That's how it works, by taking the pressure off the tendon.

Should you wear these all the time? No. The reason is similar to wearing a posture device. Once you put an external brace on, the muscles underneath switch off because they don't need to do the work. Part of the problem in tennis elbow is a weakening of the muscles and if you put a brace on you're going to get more weakness faster.

There are times when you could use them. If you are moving to a new house, you're going to be packing boxes and lifting. Stressing the tendon is going to be unavoidable. The gold standard is to have somebody else do all the lifting and moving. But if you can't and you know you're going to have to do it, the brace can be helpful to take the pressure off the tendon.

I had a client who was a plumber. He wore a brace at times when he was using his hands intensively. There are certain circumstances where it will help to protect the tendon, but it is not a long-term fix. If you can change your activities so you don't have to wear the brace, that is preferable.

8. Tape

Taping your elbow may help to reduce pain in the short term.

George et al (2019) found *"in individuals with lateral epicondylalgia, diamond deloading rigid tape may immediately improve pain and strength."* However, this is a challenging technique to apply to your own elbow, so can be helpful if you are working with an experienced therapist who can do it for you.

Cho et al (2018) showed that [kinesio] *"taping sessions produced significant improvement in pain experienced during resisted wrist extension and pain-free grip strength."* This was in sufferers who had been experiencing symptoms for at least 2 months and while the tape was on.

Eraslan et al (2018) found *"Kinesiotaping was found to be effective for decreasing pain intensity, recovering grip strength, and improving functionality in patients with lateral epicondylitis undergoing rehabilitation."* Now, the key point to note here is **"in patients with lateral epicondylitis undergoing rehabilitation."** Kinesiotape alone will NOT heal your elbow. However, it can be a useful strategy in phase 1 to help decrease pain intensity.

Giray et al (2019) also found *"kinesiotaping in addition to exercises is more effective than sham taping and exercises only in improving pain in daily activities and arm disability due to lateral epicondylitis."* Both of these two previous studies looked at patients who had suffered for less than 12 weeks.

Balevi et al (2023) also found that *"in the two weeks after Kinesio taping treatment, pain reduction persisted as a residual effect which may improve the exercise adherence and functionality."* In other words, the benefits lasted for a couple of weeks beyond the active taping period. This study focused on patients with chronic symptoms.

Hill et al (2023) found *"no benefits from applying multi-directional tape over the wrist joint."* This shows that where you put the tape is important. Seek out an experienced local practitioner to help you with this.

Kinesio tape, KT tape, and Rock Tape are all brand names of similar products. Kinesio tape was the original and first. I have unfortunately found minimal benefit for tennis elbow sufferers with the use of Kinesio tape. Although, if you have used it and found it beneficial, I would say keep using it within the parameters shown in the research.

Try not to use it all the time. If you use it too much, the skin can break down, and then you won't be able to use it. That's the biggest concern with using any kind of tape because if your skin breaks down, you're going to have to stop using it. You would also not be able to use heat or ice until the skin healed. After you've taken the tape off, rub a little milk of magnesia on the area. That can help the skin stay healthy.

If you know you're going to be doing something where you're going to be uncomfortable, put it on, but ideally, you want to get to the point where you don't have to use it. Fix it, and then you won't need to use the tape anymore.

9. Sleep

Aim for 8 hours of sleep every night, with a similar bedtime and wake up time.

Anderson et al (2023) found *"the lagged associations between sleep, and both pain and psychological distress for the chronic pain group indicate that, increased quantity of sleep predicts decreased next-day pain and psychological distress."*

Many sufferers cannot sleep at night as their elbows bother them. Sleep is essential for healing. Try and get eight hours of sleep if you can. I know it can be hard, especially if you've got kids or you have to get up early for work. Something I find helpful is using an eye mask and earplugs. They block out light and sound and I sleep much better.

If you can get a good night's sleep, you are going to heal better and faster than if you don't. Simple things like not having caffeine or alcohol before you go to bed can help. Cutting down on screen time just before you go to bed can also make a huge difference, because the blue light from the screens wakes your brain up. Once the sun's gone down, try to limit your screen time to allow your brain to go to sleep.

Try to stick to a bedtime routine. Like little kids; bath, PJs, story, bed. Their little bodies get used to that routine. Well, our big bodies like routine as well. We are creatures of habit. Try and stick to the same time going to bed every night and the same time waking up every morning. Don't shift it just because it's the weekend or a holiday but try to stick to the same routine. You're going to find you will get a better quality of sleep. If you get a better quality of sleep, you're going to feel better and heal faster.

Some people adopt the fetal position in bed. Tennis elbows don't tend to like this very much. The circulation slows down when you're in bed and that can increase irritation in that area. It tends to be more comfortable in a straight position. There are soft braces on the market that can be helpful in this situation. You can also just use a towel, rolled into a sausage shape, put it along your arm, and then hold it in place by gently wrapping a bandage around it, something that is stretchy, not tight, but just to hold it in place so that it can bend, but can't bend up fully.

The right mattress and pillow can also be immensely helpful. But which is the best? Unfortunately, there is no gold standard when it comes to mattress choice or pillow selection. I love a memory foam mattress, but many people don't. Head to the mattress store and take a good book with you. When you find a mattress that you think will work for you, settle yourself down on it and read your book for 20 minutes. Ignore the salesperson for that time and just relax. How do you feel at the end of the 20 minutes? If you feel any kind of aches and pains, that's not the mattress (or pillow) for you. But, if you feel great at the end of the 20 minutes, then you may have found a winner.

10. Pills

Take medications that have been prescribed to you by your doctor, if they appear to be helping.
Pattanittum et al (2013) reported *"We are uncertain whether non-steroidal anti-inflammatory drugs (NSAIDs) (e.g. ibuprofen, diclofenac, celecoxib) taken orally in tablet form improve pain or function because of the low quality of the evidence. NSAIDs may cause stomach, kidney or heart problems."*

Pain medications can help if you've been prescribed them and you need to take them. If you can't sleep because your elbow is very painful, you cannot heal. Your body heals when you're asleep. If you need to take pain medication before you go to bed to get a good night's sleep, that's ok to do because you need to sleep well so that you can start healing. Anti-inflammatories or muscle relaxers would be similar. If you need to use them to be comfortable, take them, if they've been prescribed to you. Ask your doctor about these. On the other hand, if you're taking a medication and it seems to make no difference to you, ask your doctor about it too.

11. Topicals

Topical anti-inflammatory gel can be helpful for the first 4 weeks. CBD lotion can also be helpful.
Pattanittum et al (2013) found in people with lateral elbow pain *"Topical NSAIDs (applied to the skin in a gel) may improve treatment success. NSAIDs applied to the skin may result in a skin rash."* They concluded that NSAID gel can be effective if used for 4 weeks.

Bussin et al (2021) found *"The regular application of topical diclofenac for Achilles tendinopathy over a 4-week period was not associated with superior clinical outcomes to that achieved with placebo."* This is good to know, as it appears to not matter what you massage over your tendon. My thought is that the action of the massage is therefore the helpful contributing factor, not necessarily the lotion/gel. More on this in phase 2.

Topical glyceryl trinitrate (GTN) treatment has previously demonstrated short-term efficacy in the treatment of lateral epicondylosis. McCallum et al (2011) found *"while GTN appears to offer short-term benefits up to 6 months in the treatment of lateral epicondylosis, at 5 years there does not appear to be significant clinical benefits when compared with patients undertaking a standard tendon rehabilitation programme alone. This is in contrast to findings of continued benefits at long-term follow-up described in the literature for patients with Achilles tendinopathy treated with GTN."* This would appear to show anatomically specific results.

Many people try creams or topicals, which you rub onto the area. An anti-inflammatory cream or gel can be helpful in the very early stage. I think sometimes the massaging, the actual moving of the soft tissues is what can be helpful. It's going to increase the circulation to the area, and that is needed.

I'm often asked about Cannabidiol or CBD. It is not my area of expertise. However, I will pass on the information that many clients find relief when using it. I've worked with patients who found CBD lotion to have dramatic effects on symptom resolution. However, it's important to remember that symptom resolution is not healing and ALL phases of the program need to be completed to achieve healing.

There is still a lot we don't know about CBD and the research is ongoing. There are so many different types of CBD. You can find the brand I recommend in the book bonuses. There are different ways of using CBD, as a tincture, edibles, and there's the topical that you put on, just like the anti-inflammatory gel.

If you are interested in trying any of these options, ask your doctor for a recommendation.

12. Nutrition

Choose a predominantly plant-based diet, which is high in protein (20–25g per meal).

Dragan et al (2020) found *"besides classical and alternative methods of treatment described in literature, it was observed that different diets are also a valid solution, due to many components with antioxidant and anti-inflammatory qualities capable of influencing chronic pain and improving quality of life."*

It is known within the fitness world that consuming protein within 30-45 minutes following a workout is beneficial to building muscle and muscle repair. Therefore, it would seem prudent to ensure that this is something to consider during rehab.

Remember that circulation brings the building blocks for healing in the bloodstream? Those building blocks for healing need to come from your nutrition; the food, the drink, the supplements you take in. Protein is what makes up the tendon and protein is needed to heal it.[28] If you are not getting enough protein in your diet, your body will take it from a source of protein in your body, which is your muscles.

Ensuring you eat a good balanced diet, making sure you're getting enough protein, calcium, all of the nutrients that you need for healing and for being healthy is going to be beneficial in your healing journey. I recommend a plant-based diet as a good go-to. You can find information about how to incorporate a plant-based diet into your life on many healthy lifestyle websites. You may want to consider a Mediterranean diet as an alternative.

13. Nutritional supplements

Taking a multivitamin containing vitamins B, C and D may be helpful, along with 10–15g of hydrolyzed collagen 30–60 minutes before exercise.

Burton et al (2023) stated, *"Nutritional supplements may have potential as an adjunctive method to standard treatment methods such as exercise, where their pain-relieving, anti-inflammatory, and structural tendon effects may augment the positive functional outcomes gained from progressive exercise rehabilitation."* Supplements can help improve the effects you get from exercise.

Hijlkema et al (2022) reported *"Individual studies showed promising clinical implications for the use of dietary supplements, particularly those containing collagen-derived peptides. However, giving any definitive dietary recommendations on the prevention and treatment of tendinopathy remains elusive."* Indeed, they went on to say that combining training and dietary supplements seems to induce better clinical and functional outcomes in tendinopathy.

Turnagöl et al (2021) found that *"intake of 10–15 g of hydrolyzed collagen per day appears to be an effective strategy for the prevention and treatment of joint, tendon, and ligament injuries."* They also found most benefit in taking it 30–60 minutes before exercise.

Jerger et al (2022) showed that *"the supplementation of specific collagen peptides combined with resistance training (RT) is associated with a greater hypertrophy in tendinous and muscular structures than RT alone in young physically active men."* It must be emphasized though, that any supplementation is just that - supplementation. You can't just take collagen and your tendon heals. It doesn't work like that. The study here shows that taking the collagen peptides improved the training effects of the exercises the subjects were doing. Supplementation can work to create the optimal environment for your tendon to heal. However, many studies agree that there is not enough evidence to support the use of specific supplements to heal tendons and more research is needed.

Noriega-González et al (2022) found *"usefulness of vitamin C (VC) in the therapeutic approach to tendinopathies. A supplementation of VC, alone or combined with other compounds, increases the production of collagen, with the consequent improvement of recovery in the patient. It is important to consider that many of the studies have been developed for injectable administration of VC in the affected area. In addition, VC deficiency is fundamentally associated with a decrease in procollagen synthesis and reduced hydroxylation of proline and lysine residues, hindering the tendon repair process. Despite this, there is no unanimity on the more efficient doses to be used. At the moment, 60 mg of VC alone or in combination with other compounds seems to be the dose mainly proposed for tendinopathy treatment. Nevertheless, when VC is taken alone as an antioxidant, higher doses have been used. Therefore, more studies have to be carried out to determine the optimal oral dose that could be useful in the resolution of this pathology. Finally, the present report is focused only on VC, but nutrition in general and exercise have to be considered together for optimal and healthy performance."*

Similar benefits have been reported with several of the B vitamins too.

At the time of writing, El-Leithy et al (2023) found *"vitamin D deficiency to be associated with lateral elbow pain."* It is hypothosized that vitamin D3 could be beneficial in the treatment of tennis elbow. This research is currently ongoing.

McCartney et al (2020) found *"There is preliminary supportive evidence for anti-inflammatory, neuroprotective, analgesic, and anxiolytic actions of CBD and the possibility it may protect against GI damage associated with inflammation and promote the healing of traumatic skeletal injuries."*

Another supplement that several clients have found useful is magnesium. These particular clients were struggling with increased muscle tension or spasm, and they found great relief by taking magnesium supplements. Ask your doctor if this could be helpful for you.

You can't just take a supplement and expect it to heal your tendon. It doesn't work like that. But if you follow the plan and do the exercises, supplements may help your tendon heal optimally.

14. Hydration

Aim for 8 glasses of water per day.

Dehydration can slow recovery. In conjunction with nutrition, we need to consider hydration. One of the major causes of pain in tennis elbow is excessive tension in the forearm muscles, which then pulls on the injured tendon. Cleary et al (2005) found *"dehydration can make muscle tension worse."* A healthy goal is to drink 8 glasses of water per day. The side effect of this will be less muscle tension, which is a great side effect to have.

When considering hydration, it's important to know that certain drinks can lead to dehydration and an increase in muscle tension. These include highly caffeinated drinks such as strong coffee, colas, and energy drinks. Alcohol is also a cause of dehydration. When you are trying to heal a tendon, consider whether you need to make small changes to your nutrition and hydration.

In their study, Hijlkema et al (2022) found that *"alcohol consumption can be a potential risk factor associated with Achilles tendinopathy and rotator cuff tears."* While there was no conclusive evidence in relation to tennis elbow. Anecdotally I have clients who know they feel their elbow pain more if they have consumed alcohol.

15. Cardio

Aim for 30 minutes of cardio exercise daily.
Tan et al (2022) found that *"aerobic exercise reduces pain sensitisation in individuals with musculoskeletal pain, such as tennis elbow."*

Öte Karaca et al (2017) found *"short-term aerobic exercise along with conventional physical therapy decreased pain sensitivity and increased aerobic capacity, with significant improvements in health-related quality of life."*

You already learned that your body is not designed to be in a sitting position all day, so what is it designed for? 10,000 years ago, there were no chairs, no phones, no laptops, no tablets. Humans were running around the fields, looking for food, chasing animals, and picking berries. Our bodies are not designed to be sitting all day in a concrete or metal box. It is not designed to be chair-shaped. It is designed to be running and exploring. Movement is essential for its well-being.

There are different forms of exercise. What I'd like you to start today is cardio exercise. "But Emma, it's my elbow. I'm not going to run around on my hands." No, you're not. But you are going to benefit from doing cardio exercise. The reason is, you need to increase your circulation. You need to get an increase in blood flow to your tendon. A really good way of increasing your circulation is cardio exercise. It can be as simple as walking and that's what I'm going to ask you to do today. I want you to do one minute of walking today. That's it. One minute. It's super simple. Nobody can say "I don't have time to go." It's one minute. You literally step out of the door and start your timer. Walk 30 seconds. Turn around and walk back. Done. Achieved. Check it off the list. Doing cardio exercise is going to increase your circulation and kickstart the healing process.

Are you going to stick with one minute every day? No, you're going to build up slowly. The ideal is to build up every single day, no days off. You're doing cardio exercise so that your tendon can heal. You need to do the cardio exercise every single day and ideally increase the duration by a minute each day. So, tomorrow you're going to do two minutes, the day after, three minutes, the day after, four minutes. Slowly building up over time until you get to 30 minutes. It will take you a month from today to get there, which is why you're starting today because if you start next week, it's going to be a month from then. Start today, with one minute of cardio exercise.

If you are used to exercising, start 30 minutes of daily cardio exercise today.

You can find a Cardio Calendar here:

http://bit.ly/TE-bookbonuses

16. Relaxation

Practice progressive relaxation before you go to sleep every night.

The muscles in your forearm, neck, upper traps, and around your shoulder are likely tight. They need to relax. Progressive relaxation is something that can help with that.

Progressive relaxation is a guided relaxation that is perfect for the bedtime routine. It's progressive, in that you start at the top of your body and work your way down. Or you can start from your toes and work your way up. But the goal is to get relaxation of all the different muscle groups. I tend to start from my toes and work my way up. I say this because I use this strategy myself. If I can't fall asleep, I use progressive relaxation to help relax my body and allow me to get to sleep. So, I suggest that you do this at nighttime when you get into bed. If you fall asleep before you've finished, perfect. You don't get more relaxed than that.

This is how I go through my progressive relaxation:

- Lie on your back in a comfortable position, and close your eyes. Start with your toes. Curl your toes as tightly as you can and hold the contraction tight, tight, tight, tight, tight, holding it for 10 seconds. Then release and literally just relax.

- Then pull your toes back towards you as far as you can, hold them tight, tight, tight, tight, tight, tight, tight release.

- Then move on to your ankles. Point your feet down, as far as they can go. Hold it tight, tight, tight, tight, tight, for 10 seconds, then release.

- Now pull your feet back and hold it tight, tight, tight, tight, tight, tight, tight, for 10 seconds and release.

- Then push your knees down. Push them as straight as they'll go. Tight, tight, tight, tight, tight, tight, tight, really tighten those muscles and drop. It's a release, a drop.

- Squeeze your glutes, your butt muscles (bum if you're in the UK). 10-second hold. Release.

- Pull your tummy muscles in as much as you can. Pull, pull, pull, pull, pull, pull, pull, pull, relax.

- Pull your shoulders back to the bed. Press them back behind you. Squeeze, squeeze, squeeze, squeeze, release.

- Now, depending on how your arm feels, you can either do the arm exercises or not. If you are going to do them, straighten your elbows as much as you can. Generally, that's okay for most people. If it's not okay for you, don't do it. Press your elbows as straight as you can. Press, press, press, press, press, press, press 10 seconds and release.

- And then make tight fists. If that doesn't feel okay for you, don't do it. 10-second hold, then release.

- Spread your fingers out wide. Hold it for 10 seconds. Squeeze, squeeze, squeeze, release.

- Now take your shoulders up towards your ears. Tight, tight, tight, tight, tight, tight, tight, tight, tight. Release.
- Press your head back into the pillow. Press, press, press, press, press, press, press, press, release.
- Now we get to the face ones and these are my favorite. Screw your face up into a frown as tightly as you can, tight, tight, tight, release,
- Then a big wide smile, tight, tight, tight, tight, tight, tight, tight, relax, and then just drop and rest.
- You will literally feel your body just sinking and melting into the bed. It feels fantastic to do.

Well done! That's your first progressive relaxation session completed.

You can find this in audio format in the book bonuses here:

http://bit.ly/TE-bookbonuses

The theory behind progressive relaxation is that when you do a maximum contraction of a muscle, it is followed by maximum relaxation of the same muscle. That's the way the muscles work. You're going to get full relaxation of the muscle. But it needs to be comfortable. If it's not comfortable in any way, don't do it and move on to do a different body part.

I start from my toes and work my way up. If you want to start from the top of your head and work your way down, that's completely fine. If you fall asleep before you finish, brilliant, you are nice and relaxed. Sometimes you might need to go through it two or three times, and that's ok too.

Start tonight. When you get into bed, go through your progressive relaxation. You don't have to listen to a video. You can go through it in your head. Although, sometimes listening to something can be helpful to really cue you into what you should be feeling as you learn this new technique. It's training you how to do it.

17. Visualization

Build up to 5–10 minutes of visualization per day.
For visualization, you're using your imagination. You're really using your brain to visualize things in intense detail. Athletes use visualization often throughout their training. Research has shown that strength can be gained by visualization alone.[31]

I was introduced to visualization as a young gymnast. I can remember our coach got us all to think about a teacup. At the time we would snigger to each other. What the heck is he talking about? Think of a teacup! But that is how he would start our visualization sessions. Then we would visualize ourselves going through the gymnastic moves that we were learning. You immerse yourself in the experience and imagine yourself performing the movement flawlessly, over and over again.

Anybody who plays any sport can use visualization. It is effective even for people who are not sports people. Musicians can visualize playing their instruments. It works even for people who just have one particular task that they want to accomplish pain-free. Maybe it's picking up a bottle of water, picking up your cup of coffee, or picking up a gallon of milk. You can use visualization to help achieve it.

Visualization is an incredibly powerful tool working on the brain. It tricks the brain into thinking that your body can do that particular activity pain-free. For example, I had a client who was a softball player, and she couldn't play because her elbow was injured. She visualized pitching, throwing and batting every day in intense detail. You've got to use all of your senses with visualization. You've got to see it, hear it, smell it, touch it, taste it. You've got to be totally in the moment.

Start visualization today. Ideally, you want to be somewhere quiet. You're not going to do this when you're driving or in a busy work area or with kids screaming in the background. You want to be in a quiet place so you can focus on what you're doing. You can do it lying down, or sitting if that's more comfortable. Close your eyes, so that you can immerse yourself in the moment.

Think of the softball player who's visualizing throwing. She is going to feel the ball in her hand. She's going to feel where her arm is, though, she's not physically moving. She's resting in the same position, but she is feeling it as though she is there. She feels the sun on her face. She takes a step forward and cocks her arm back and then she throws the ball and she throws it perfectly. The thing about visualization is you are not moving whilst you're visualizing. This is not going to be detrimental at all to your elbow, as you're not doing the motion physically.

What visualization does is reinforce the neural pathways that your body switches on when you do that particular movement. Let me explain what I mean by that. A neural pathway is the message that the brain sends to your muscles to say, switch on in this way, to perform that task. Now, when you do something so many times, it becomes automatic. This is the basis of motor learning.

Motor learning can be explained by the following. Imagine a little kid learning to ride a bike and they're trying to take the training wheels off (stabilizers if you're in the UK). They're trying and trying and they keep falling off because they haven't got the correct neural pathway set yet. Their brain hasn't learned how to send the correct messages. "Which muscles am I switching on to balance and pedal and steer and stay up?" It doesn't know yet. So, they practice, and practice and they fall off, and each time they're getting new information and new input.

All of a sudden, they get it, and off they go, with the biggest smile on their face. That's motor learning in action. They didn't know how to do a task and all of a sudden, they did. What's happened is they found the correct neural pathway. That is the message that the brain sends down to the muscles and the joints to say, move in this way so you can stay up on that bike and you can keep going.

When they get it and they're doing it, they are strengthening that neural pathway. They strengthen it each time they perform the movement. What visualization does is strengthen that neural pathway, without you moving. Your brain will send the messages to the muscles and the joints, to fire in that way, to move in that way. When you make that perfect pitch, when you throw that perfect ball, when you hit that perfect shot, whatever it may be, the brain is going to strengthen those neural pathways.

Right now, you can't play tennis. You can't play golf. You can't play the drums. You can't play the guitar. You're not lifting. You're not picking your kids up. You're not working out or whatever else you may be prevented from doing. You want to make sure you don't lose the neural pathways associated with those activities because if you don't use them, you lose them. You don't completely forget how to do the movement, you know you can always ride a bike, but it's probably not as good as if you'd been practicing it the whole time.

You want to keep the neural pathways sharp and strong so that when you can get back to hitting a ball, throwing a ball, working out, playing the violin, or whatever it is you're going to do, those neural pathways are ready for you to do that activity. That's what visualization will do for you. I challenge you to do visualization for 5 minutes today.

Recap

To recap, you've got a lot of fun stuff to try today:

- Staying pain-free
- Heat – 10 minutes out of every hour
- Ice – only if you need it
- Keeping good posture and ergonomics
- Different types of brace (don't do it, if you don't need to)
- Pills or creams (again, don't use them if you don't need them)
- Get a good night's sleep – around 8 hours is optimal
- Good nutrition and hydration – protein at every meal and snack
- Cardio exercise – build up to 30 minutes daily
- Progressive relaxation – when you go to bed
- Visualization – 5 minutes

Do you see how all of these different components matter? Can you imagine just doing ultrasound on your elbow and not doing the rest of it? It's no wonder people don't get better. If you do all these things, you are going to feel so much better.

These strategies make up the bulk of phase one. Phase one is where you're really feeling the symptoms, where you're really uncomfortable. These self-help strategies will help you set your healing foundation. Miss it out and you've got a shaky base to build from.

The next chapter adds a few additional strategies for people who have had tennis elbow for 3 months or longer. If this is you, please read on. If you've been suffering for less than 3 months, please feel free to skip Chapter 7 and jump ahead to Chapter 8.

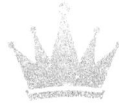

Additional Phase 1 Self-Help Strategies If You've Had Pain For Longer Than 3 Months

Phase 1 Goals

- Reduce symptoms
- Begin to normalize the nervous system
- Start sport-specific visualization

Additional Phase 1 Strategies

1. Nutritional supplements - Lion's Mane
2. Forest bathing
3. Calm the nervous system
4. Breathwork
5. Meditation
6. Tai Chi

1. Nutritional supplements – Lion's Mane

Ask your doctor about taking Lion's Mane daily if you have nerve symptoms.

Sabaratnam et al (2013) found *"the studies show that selected mushrooms do have neurotrophic properties that can be beneficial to humans. Regular consumption may promote nerve and brain health. This is particularly useful during injury."*

Li et al (2018) found that *"results have indicated that administration of **H. erinaceus mycelia** (Lions Mane) enriched with its active compounds can promote functional recovery and enhance nerve regeneration in rats with neuropathic pain."*

Lion's Mane is a supplement derived from the Lion's Mane mushroom and is marketed as a memory enhancer or brain booster. I first heard about this supplement a few years ago, when I was working with a client who had had a severe injury to his shoulder causing nerve damage to his arm. He is a yoga instructor and as such was very keen on natural remedies. He made the fastest recovery from a nerve injury that I have ever seen, and he put it down to his taking Lion's Mane.

Since working with him, and witnessing the amazing recovery he made, I have recommended this supplement to clients who describe nerve symptoms. This may be tingling, pins and needles, numbness, or pain, that I recognize as being nerve in origin, and many seem to benefit from taking Lion's Mane. If you are unsure whether this would be a good choice for you, ask your doctor about it.

2. Forest bathing

Spend 20 minutes once per week out in nature, or do your daily 30-minute cardio outside.

Li (2010) stated, *"In Japan, a forest bathing trip, called "Shinrinyoku" in Japanese, is a short, leisurely visit to a forest and is regarded as being similar to natural aromatherapy. A forest bathing trip involves visiting a forest for relaxation and recreation while breathing in volatile substances, called phytoncides (wood essential oils), which are antimicrobial volatile organic compounds derived from trees, such as α-pinene and limonene. Forest bathing has now become a recognized relaxation and/or stress management activity in Japan."*

Wen et al (2019) demonstrated that *"forest bathing activities might have the following merits: remarkably improving cardiovascular function, hemodynamic indexes, neuroendocrine indexes, metabolic indexes, immunity and inflammatory indexes, antioxidant indexes, and electrophysiological indexes; significantly enhancing people's emotional state, attitude, and feelings towards things, physical and psychological recovery, and adaptive behaviors; and obvious alleviation of anxiety and depression."* Can you imagine if a pill did all of these things? It would be the most prescribed drug of all time.

Weston-Green et al (2021) found *"evidence supporting the health benefits of forest volatile organic compounds rich in terpenes such as pinene, linalool, limonene and caryophyllene, could provide an alternative approach to positive outcomes for well-being. There is some evidence that these terpenes provide therapeutic efficacy similar to existing commercial medications for several indications, including analgesics, anti-inflammatories ... with fewer adverse effects e.g., sedation and motor impairment."*

Good nutrition, adequate sleep, proper hydration and being outside and seeing green things, are all essential for our body to work most efficiently and effectively. You've already heard about most of the things mentioned above, but what about the "being outside and seeing green things" part? This is a hugely underutilized strategy that is essential for our body's well-being. If someone has been experiencing pain for longer than 3 months, they have chronic pain. Chronic pain produces biochemical and anatomical changes in the brain.[25] These changes can be reversed by "rebooting" the brain.[29] Getting out into nature can do this. This is why I advise you to do 30 minutes of cardio exercise every day, **preferably outside**, so that you can see green things like plants, trees, flowers, and grass

This may sound a little bit woo-woo, but if you immerse yourself in nature, you can reboot your brain. If you have chronic pain, your nervous system is hypersensitized in a state of fight or flight. It is essential to break that cycle. Getting into nature can help to do that. By rebooting your brain, you calm the nervous system down. The nervous system is going to stop sending all of those pain messages and you can start your healing journey. If you don't do that, you're going to struggle to heal.

If you are used to exercising, start 30 minutes of cardio exercise today, preferably outside. If you live somewhere that is very hot, choose your time of day. Go first thing in the morning, or go last thing at night, if that feels better for you. Don't go out in the heat of the middle of the day. If you live somewhere that is very wet, don't go out in the rain. Choose your time and choose your place.

Heart health and brain health are intricately intertwined. Take cardio exercise, before today, you may have just associated cardio exercise with physical fitness. But cardio exercise plays a huge role in mental fitness too. It makes sense really when you consider the increase in circulation you get with cardio exercise. You get an increase in blood flow to the muscles and tendons. But you also get that increase in circulation to the brain.

There are other strategies I advocate regarding the mind-body connection. You may feel that these are so similar that you just choose to do one. However, you would be missing out on the distinct and important benefits each one brings to the healing of tennis elbow. I encourage you to add them all to allow you to heal in the fastest time possible.

3. Calm the nervous system

Join the next Empowered Relief® class to calm your nervous system.

Empowered Relief® is an evidence-based, single-session pain class that rapidly equips patients with pain management skills including using breathwork to transition from a Pain or Stress Response to a Relaxation Response.

If persistent pain gets in the way of living the life you want, I hope you will join me for the next Empowered Relief® class.

Empowered Relief® is a skills-based, single-session training developed by pain psychologists at Stanford University and taught exclusively by certified instructors. This live, virtual class rapidly equips attendees with pain management skills to address ongoing pain that interferes with your quality of life. Research shows that attendees experience lasting benefits from Empowered Relief®, including reduced pain intensity, better sleep, lower stress, and more.

You will walk away from this 2-hour training with:

- A deeper understanding of the neuroscience behind pain
- A robust set of skills that you can count on to decrease the ways chronic pain negatively affects your daily life
- An audio file combining binaural beats with guided meditation
- An individualized plan you can turn to for pain relief

From the comfort of your home, join me for just 2 hours to learn simple yet impactful strategies that you can use right away to manage your chronic pain.

Learn more and sign up for the next class, here:

https://www.tenniselbowqueen.com/empoweredrelief

4. Breathwork

Spend a few minutes focusing on deep breathing each day.

Breathwork can be incredibly powerful in calming the nervous system. Breathing is an essential action our bodies need to stay healthy. But what about the quality of the breathing? I'm not talking about the quality of the air that you're breathing, although that too is super important. I'm talking about the actual quality of the inhaling and exhaling that you are doing. Have you ever thought about it? Do it now. Just stop reading for a second and take a couple of breaths.

Do you feel the air going deep down into the base of your lungs, or is it staying up at the top of the lungs? Does your tummy fill outwards as you take a deep breath in, dropping gently as you breathe out?

This motion, as automatic as it is, can become less than efficient. If this happens, the breaths tend to become less deep and more shallow. The air at the base of the lungs may become stagnant and as such, how can it promote optimum exchange of oxygen into the body? Poor posture or prolonged sitting are two of the things that can negatively affect good breathing.

Start practicing good breathing techniques today. Diaphragmatic breathing encourages the optimum use of the diaphragm, which is the major muscle involved in breathing. Sit comfortably in a chair and rest your hands on your belly. As you breathe in, feel the tummy gently expanding outward. As you breathe out, feel the tummy gently sink back in. If you don't feel your tummy moving as you breathe, it may be that you are breathing at the top of your lungs and you need to practice getting the air down to the bases.

5. Meditation

Spend 5 minutes following a guided meditation today.

Meditation is something that is becoming more mainstream. I always used to think it was a little bit woo-woo, and it wasn't really my thing, but the more I learn about it, the more I realize we all should be doing this. It is so good for our brains and brain biochemistry.

The reasons for meditation are twofold. One, it helps with relaxation. You become aware of any tension your body might be holding. That's the physical aspect. The other side is you are resting your brain. This is helpfull for chronic pain sufferers to break the cycle of their pain.

Chronic pain changes the biochemistry in your brain and it changes the anatomy of your brain. The reason being is that the nervous system is sending pain messages to the brain. The nervous system is sending pain, pain, pain, pain, and the brain is essentially saying okay, what should I do about it? That goes on and on and on. This process changes the chemicals in your brain, and it changes the anatomy. However, these changes are reversible. Meditation allows normalizing of the biochemistry in the brain.[30]

Start doing meditation so that you are giving your brain a rest, and calming down the nervous system. There are some fantastic, guided meditations available. Calm is an app that you can use for guided meditation. Headspace is another one. You can access guided meditation on YouTube. I really love Deepak Chopra's guided meditations. You can find him on YouTube and Facebook. I challenge you to start meditation today, just 5 minutes can help.

I know meditation and visualization sound similar, but they work in very different ways. In meditation, you are giving the brain a rest. You're not thinking about anything. In visualization, you are working and strengthening the brain.

6. Tai Chi

Do 5 minutes of Tai Chi daily.
Hall et al (2017) found that *"tai chi was more effective than no treatment or usual care at short term on pain."*

Kong et al (2016) reported *"Tai Chi as a viable complementary and alternative medicine for chronic pain conditions."*

I recommend 5 minutes of Tai Chi daily. You'll see as we progress through the program that this activity will morph into more sport-specific or activity-specific movements.

Phase 1 Recap

To recap:

- Nutritional supplementation – Lion's Mane
- Forest bathing (get out into nature)
- Breathwork to counteract the pain and stress responses
- Meditation
- Tai Chi

Can you see how these additional components fit into your healing strategy? Can you imagine just doing one of these things and not doing the rest? If you do all these things, you are going to feel so much better. These strategies make up phase one. Phase one is where you're really feeling the symptoms, where you're really uncomfortable. These self-help strategies will set your healing foundation. Miss it out and you've got a shaky base to build from.

There's a daily checklist of all the phase 1 and 2 self-help strategies later in the book.

Let's move on to phase 2.

TENNIS ELBOW QUEEN

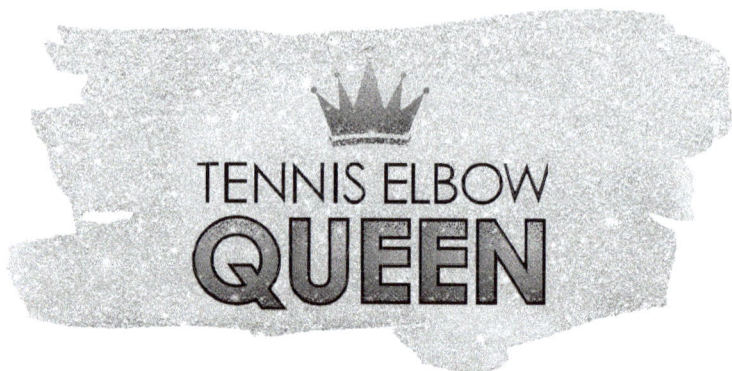

"I was able to start back playing softball and my arm feels fine! Thank you so much for taking care of me when everyone else said they couldn't. You are a miracle worker!"

CC 18

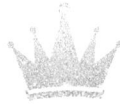

CHAPTER 8

Phase 2
Normalize Muscle Tension

The following strategies ADD IN with what you are already doing from phase 1. Don't stop phase 1 strategies when you start phase 2. They combine seamlessly together. You'll find a checklist for all the phase 1 and 2 strategies at the end of the book. If you've had tennis elbow symptoms for less than 3 months you may only need the first stretch, or maybe the first 5 strategies. If you've suffered for longer than 3 months, you'll likely need them all.

Phase 2 Goals
- Normalize the soft tissues
- Regain range of motion
- Continue to calm the nervous system
- Add non-irritating activity-specific movements

Phase 2 Strategies

1. Stretches
2. Trigger point release
3. Soft tissue massage
4. Neck retractions
5. Knee rolling
6. Shoulder rolls
7. Yoga
8. Activity-specific movements

1. Getting soft for the soft tissues

Soft tissues, like muscles, accommodate the stresses and strains put through them. For example, if you spend all day sitting, the muscles and soft tissues at the front of your hips are in a shortened position. Stay there for a prolonged period of time and the soft tissues will shorten. Muscle tension or spasm can often be part of the problem. So, what is muscle spasm, and what causes it?

Muscle spasm, cramp, or Charlie Horse, all describe the same thing, a muscle getting so tight that it can't switch itself off or relax. If you've ever experienced this, you know how painful it can be. You may need to jump out of bed at night if you get a cramp in your leg.

Why does it happen? Firstly, the body may cause a "splinting" effect to protect an injured area. The pain you feel can lead to an increase in muscle tension. Hold your injured arm in a poor posture or position and your muscle tension will go up. Additionally, excessive muscle use, such as if you've spent two hours pulling weeds, or painting the garden fence, can also increase muscle tension.

A hyper-firing nerve is one of the scenarios that doesn't often get addressed. The hyper-firing nerve or hypersensitized nervous system can be a big factor in tennis elbow's stubbornness to heal, partly due to the fact that it can trigger an increase in muscle tension. This is why many of the strategies recommended in phase 1, address the nervous system. Has it ever been suggested to you to use meditation, progressive relaxation, and nature to reboot your brain, to heal your elbow? This is what makes this solution so different to anything else.

Dehydration was mentioned earlier as a situation that can delay healing. It can also increase muscle tension and increase your pain. A lack of salt can occasionally cause problems with normal muscle function, including excessive muscle tension. I discussed supplements that clients have found useful for this issue in the nutrition section in Chapter 6.

2. We should learn from the animals

Every morning when my little dog gets up, he is desperate to come and say "Hi" to me, and his little tail looks like it's going to wag off. However, he doesn't jump out of his bed to come and give me kisses until he has stretched his front legs, and then stretches one of his back legs, and then his other back leg. Then and only then, will he come and say "Hi" to his mama. No one has told animals to stretch when they first get up, they do it instinctively.

Stretches can be very effective as long as you're doing the right ones. Stretch it out safely. Stretches should always feel comfortable. They should never illicit, what I call the "Pain Face", you know the one that you pull when you've had a really deep tissue massage, or when you step on a piece of Lego (parents, you feel me?). Stretches should never feel painful. It's ok to feel a stretch sensation, but not pain.

Heat can be really helpful before you stretch too, unless it's within the first three days of a fresh injury in which case you would just use ice. However, a heating pad, a hot shower or a hot towel can be really helpful at increasing circulation to the area. As you learned in chapter 6, you want to get fresh blood to the area as the circulation brings the building blocks for healing that your body needs when it's trying to heal an injury, and heat can also relax tight muscles. If you've got muscle spasm around the elbow or the neck and shoulders, that can be uncomfortable.

Stretching for flexibility helps to regain any range of motion that may have been lost. Sometimes, if you have an injury, you don't want to move that area. If you don't move an area for a while, that area is going to get stiff. This is because your body adapts to the stresses and strains that you're putting through it. If you're not moving a joint through its full range of motion, the soft tissues around it will shorten to accommodate. While this process in itself is normal, your tissues are accommodating to everything you do, be it marathon training, sitting at a desk all day, or limiting the use of your arm as it's painful. A lack of range of motion is not normal.

Stretching can be a great way to regain the range of motion. Ensure you're holding the stretch comfortably and maintain the stretch statically for 30 seconds. Lots of research has been done on the effectiveness of stretching. If you hold a stretch for less than 30 seconds, that's a good warm-up stretch, but it isn't going to increase your flexibility or your range of motion. However, holding a stretch for at least 30 seconds will lead to an increase in your range and flexibility.[32]

30 seconds will feel like a long time. Time yourself to ensure you are holding it long enough. If you can tolerate

holding a stretch for 30 seconds, then you only need to do it once. Repeating it over and over won't gain you any more benefit. However, repeating the stretch often throughout the day, preferably after the heat can lead to increased flexibility and reduced symptoms.

3. Joints are designed to move

All joints like to move as it's what they are designed to do. Indeed, joints get their nutrition through movement. Joint surfaces are covered with cartilage, which reduces friction and allows the joint surfaces to move smoothly over each other. When the joints move through their full range of motion, the joint fluid which bathes the joint surfaces, is squeezed out of the cartilage, giving nutrition to the joint. (Think about pressing a fountain pen onto a piece of paper and the ink flowing out.) Therefore, if joints don't go through their full range of motion regularly, they get less nutrition, which in turn can lead to the joint becoming stiffer. Takahashi et al (2021) found that *"disuse of a joint can lead to thinning of the articular cartilage."* This is seen in the development of osteoarthritis of joints.

If a joint starts to stiffen up, you start to move even less, which leads to less nutrition and thinner cartilage, which feels bad. Therefore, you move even less, and so on and so on. Takes us back to the animals that stretch every time they get out of bed.

For these reasons, my Comprehensive Elbow Pain Relief Program includes 15 different stretches and soft tissue techniques to work on normalizing the soft tissues in Phase 2. In this Chapter, you'll learn the simple stretch you need to heal your tennis elbow. Then we'll dive deeper into the other stretches that you'll need if your tennis elbow is chronic.

Wrist extensor stretch

This is the most important stretch, and it's for the wrist extensor muscles. These are generally tight when you have tennis elbow because the tendon is uncomfortable. As the muscles tense up, they pull on the tendon and it becomes even more uncomfortable. So, it's important that you stretch the muscles out.

The best way to do that is to hold your arm out in front of you with your palm down towards the floor. Make sure your shoulder stays down. Don't let it creep up to your ear. Point your fingers down towards the floor bending at the wrist. Put the thumb of your unaffected hand into the palm of your affected hand, fingers on the back of the hand, and pull towards you.

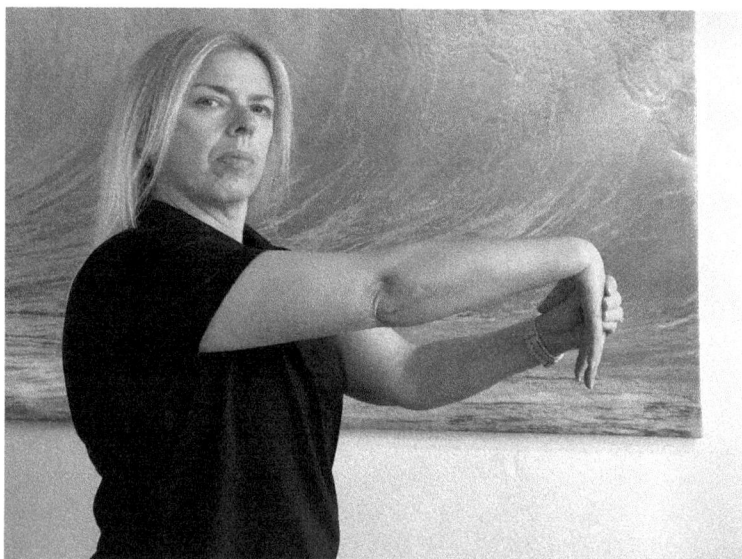

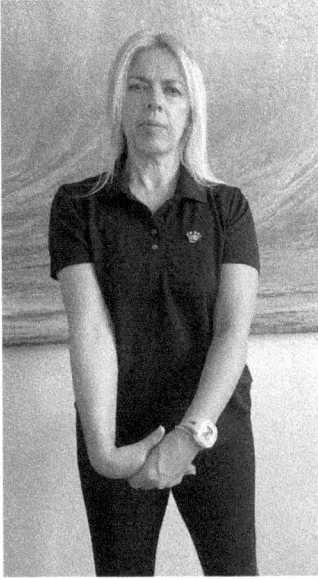

Once, you have a nice stretch through the forearm muscles by being in this position, you can allow your arm to rest down in front of your body. Hold this stretch for 30 seconds. It needs to be comfortable. No pain face. If it is too intense, ease out of the stretch slightly and hold it where it feels good for you.

Ideally, do the heat first, and then stretch it out. This one needs to be done at least 3x a day – morning, afternoon, evening, or breakfast, lunch, and dinner. Many people will stretch regularly during the day because it feels so good. You can do this sitting at your desk. It's a super easy stretch to do.

If you've been feeling your elbow for less than 3 months, you may not be feeling tension or tightness in other areas and you can skip the next sections. However, if you are feeling tight, add in the following strategies.

Trigger point release

Trigger pointing or trigger point release is a soft tissue treatment technique that you can do yourself using your fingers or a specific trigger point release tool. This technique can be used through the forearm, biceps, triceps, upper traps - any muscle that feels tight.

Start by feeling through the forearm muscles. What you're feeling for, is an area of tenderness or tension. You might feel a little tighter in one spot. When you find it put a firm pressure on it. Just enough to blanch your fingernail. Practice that on your hand; put your finger on your hand, and press just so that the fingernail changes color. You'll see it's not a lot of pressure You're not digging in. It's a light pressure. Then just hold it; you're not going to massage or move. Hold it for 60 seconds.

This should not hurt your fingers. If it's starting to hurt your fingers, you're pushing too hard. Ease off a little so that you're not pushing as deeply. Just maintain the pressure. Just hold it. You might feel like you've taken some tension off. But you probably didn't. It's the muscle relaxing.

Sometimes, you may feel the muscle twitching as you hold the pressure. That's called fasciculation. The muscle doesn't know whether to switch on or off. Just keep the pressure on. You can choose to do this on both arms. The only caveat to that is that when you're doing the opposite side it doesn't affect the elbow that has symptoms.

When you've done your trigger point release in one spot. You can then search for a different area. Because the spot you've just worked on has relaxed, there may well now be a different spot that you need to work on to relax too. Just repeat it in the same way; a 60-second hold of the firm pressure.

This technique is more effective after heat or when your body temperature is up. Use times throughout the day when your body temperature is up a little higher than normal, to bring the muscle tension down. You may find as you repeat this through the day, that it's not the same spot every time. That's normal because as you release one area, another area may well be tighter. Just work on what you feel. Wherever it feels the tightest that's the spot that you're going to work on.

For somebody who's not had tennis elbow for very long, their muscles may not have become too tight, and they may respond quickly to the trigger point release. For somebody who's had tennis elbow for much longer, the muscles have become tight and this is their new "normal". You might find that after you've done the heat and the trigger point release, the muscle will tighten back up. So, then you need to do it again. You need to do this consistently. The more you can do it, the more you're going to get relaxation and the quicker you'll feel better.

Soft tissue massage

This is the phase where you can use soft tissue massage. You can use any oil or lotion that you already have around the house, you don't need anything special. Start by gently rubbing around the elbow but avoid the sore spot of the tendon as you don't want to irritate it. You can work on the forearm muscles, biceps, and triceps muscles of the upper arm too. Even the upper traps can benefit from some soft tissue work. The key to this is to keep it comfortable for the muscles and your hands.

Neck retractions (aka chin tucks)

I know it seems weird, a neck exercise to help you heal your elbow, but it works. For this exercise, lie down on your back, with your knees bent up and feet flat on the bed.

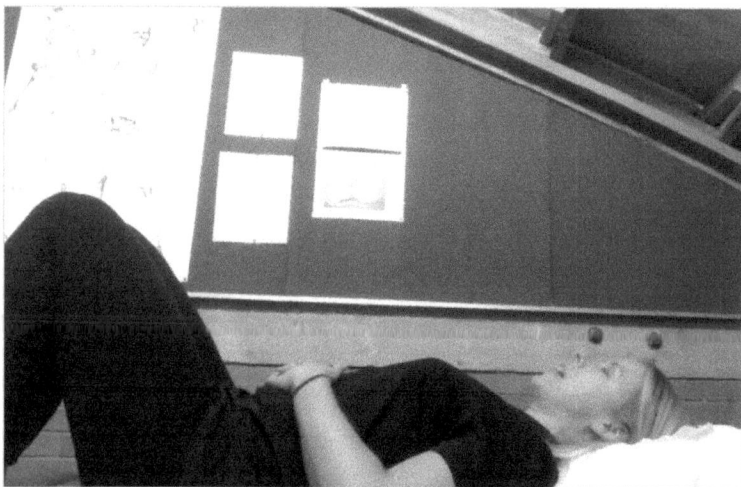

Gently press the back of your head into the pillow. Use a thin flat pillow, if it feels comfortable. You don't need to hold this position, just get there and release.

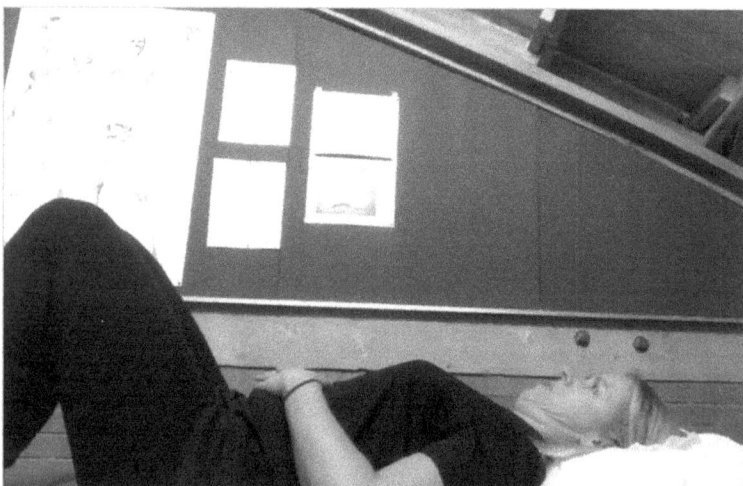

Remember that all exercises should feel comfortable, so you may need to start with a smaller movement and work up to a full range of motion. Do 10 of these exercises, 3 times per day. You can watch a video of me teaching this exercise and going into the reasons why I use it in the book bonuses:

http://bit.ly/TE-bookbonuses

Upper traps stretch

I love this stretch too. It feels so good! This stretch targets the muscle between the head and the shoulder. These are our stress muscles. 10 minutes in traffic and these tighten up. If you are feeling pain, these will tighten up. If they are tight, they can pull on the connective tissue that travels up and over the top of your head causing tension headaches. They can also pull on your neck leading to reduced range of motion or stiffness. If they pull on your shoulder, that can cause soreness, but it can also squeeze on the nerves, which can irritate them, particularly if they are hypersensitive.

Take your chin down towards your chest and then take your ear down to your shoulder.

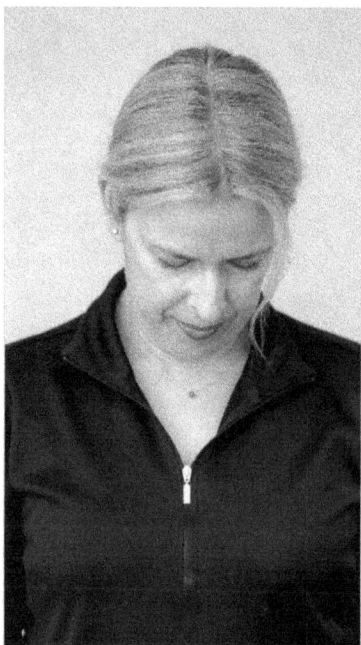

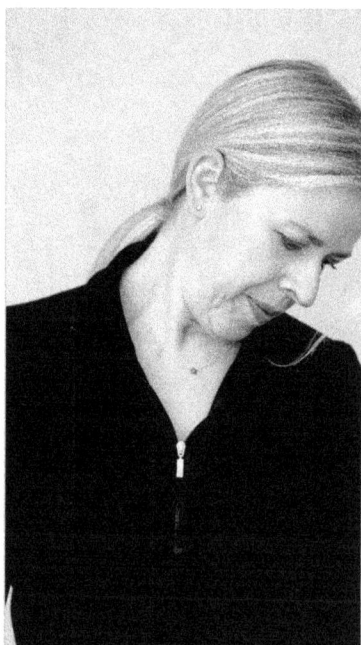

You should feel a stretch in the muscle between the neck and the shoulder. Hold it, comfortably, for 30 seconds. Repeat on the other side. You might find that the affected side is tighter, so stretch it again.

Other stretches

You may need other stretches too depending on how long you've had symptoms. I recommend you see an experienced healthcare provider who can check out other muscles that may be involved. You may need to stretch out your pecs, biceps, triceps, wrist flexors, and even the wrist joints themselves.

Knee rolling

This is one of my all-time favorite exercises. If you add this to your daily routine, before you get out of bed each morning, you will start to be able to get out of bed with less back stiffness. It works by essentially "oiling the joints", increasing the circulation, and stretching out the muscles and soft tissues. But the reason it helps heal your elbow is that it gently mobilizes the nervous system, encouraging good circulation to and within the nervous system and helping to calm it down.

Do this first thing in the morning and last thing at night. Lie down on your back with your knees bent up so your feet are flat on the bed.

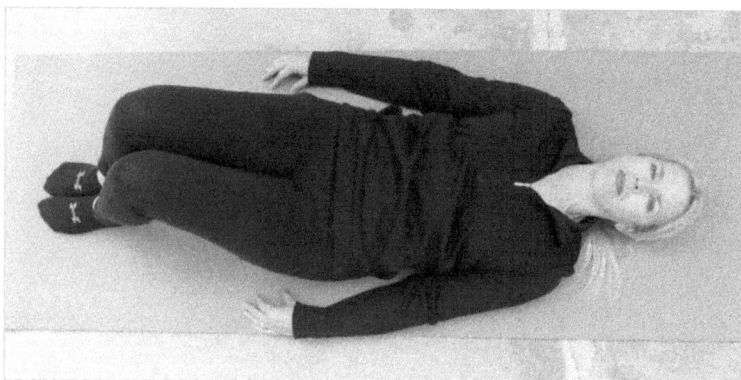

You're just going to let your knees roll from side to side, but your feet don't lift up.

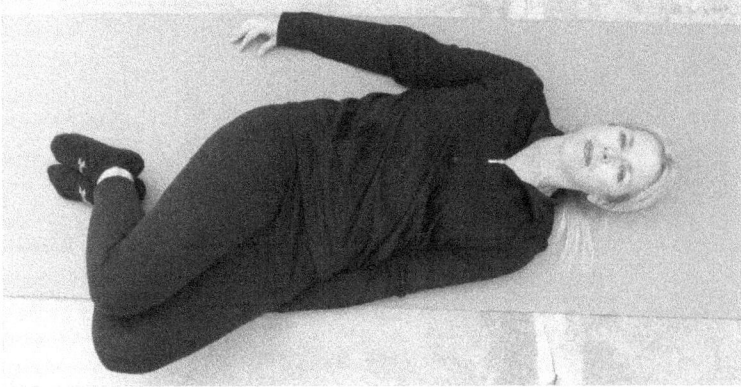

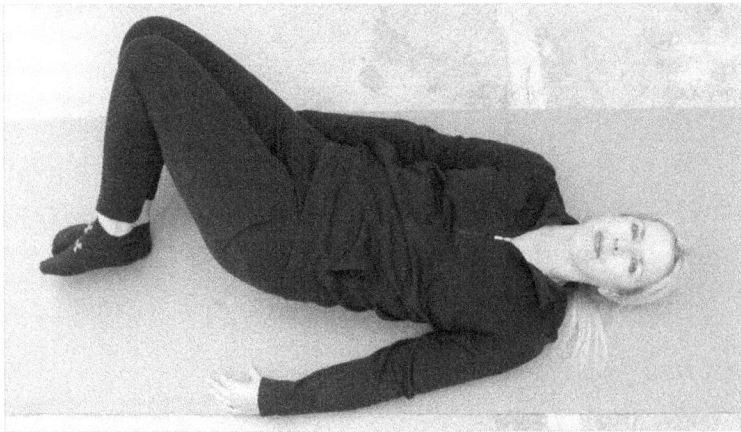

This is not a core exercise. It's not a strengthening exercise. It's a mobility exercise, and you're just rolling your knees from side to side.

Shoulder rolls

This is another fave. There are quite a few in this phase, I have to admit. It's probably because stretching is just so good for us!

It's another super simple exercise, and also a nerve mobilization exercise. Take your shoulders up towards your ears and then roll them back and down. Rotating in this direction also encourages good posture. Whereas, rotating the shoulders forward and down, tends to pull the body into a poor posture position.

Aim for 10 reps, three times daily, but stop if you feel nerve symptoms like tingling, pins and needles, numbness or pain.

4. Yoga

Phase 2 progresses the slow, upright movements of Tai Chi, into the more intense poses of yoga for the reasons given below, plus the natural progression of the intensity of the movements. If you are new to yoga, you may want to start with beginner's yoga or even chair yoga. If you already practice, feel free to increase what you are doing or add daily short sessions at home.

Basu-Ray (2021) stated *"Yoga has been found to have inhibited every baneful effect of stress. In fact, it also changes the neuronal circuits that potentiate pathological changes."* In simple terms, yoga can change the nerve pathways that lead to pathology or negative changes.

Woodyard (2011) showed that *"yogic practices enhance muscular strength and body flexibility, promote and improve respiratory and cardiovascular function, promote recovery from and treatment of addiction, reduce stress, anxiety, depression, and chronic pain, improve sleep patterns, and enhance overall well-being and quality of life."* So why are we all not doing it?

McCall (2007) stated *"Yoga encourages one to relax, slow the breath, and focus on the present, shifting the balance from the sympathetic nervous system and the flight-or-fight response to the parasympathetic system and the relaxation response."* So yoga has been shown to calm the nervous system. They also showed that *"The beneficial effects of yoga have been shown to be dose specific."* That is, the more you do, the more you benefit.

5. Activity-specific movements

This is when you can start adding in activity-specific movements. However, you are not going to be holding anything in your hands, no racket or club for example. But you can test out some super slow movements. Think about the Tai Chi that you started in phase 1 – the slow, rhythmical movements - and combine that with movements you would do in your chosen sport. Maybe you practice a super slow serve motion or try a golf swing movement. Remember, that you still need to keep yourself 100% comfortable. This is NOT the time to start pushing into pain. However, if you find you can comfortably complete all the movements you would do in your sport or activity, in slo-mo, then you can start to increase the speed until you hit normal motion.

Do NOT add anything in your hands yet. You've got to build up your strength. Talking of which, let's continue on to phase 3.

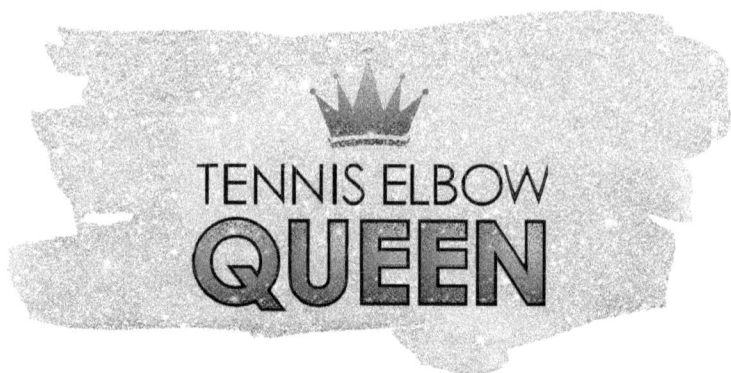

TENNIS ELBOW
QUEEN

66 Emma is a wealth of information! I NEVER heard such detailed information. Thank you! 99

RB 54

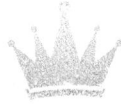

CHAPTER 9

Phase 3
The Magic of Strengthening

Phase 3 Goals

- Strengthening to heal
- Forearm strengthening starts once the muscle tension of the forearm has normalized
- Regain proprioception
- Activity-specific movements intensify

Phase 3 Strategies

1. Heavy load eccentrics
2. Core
3. Upper quadrant strengthening
4. Proprioception exercises
5. Activity-specific progressions

Once you have decreased the muscle tension in the forearm, you are ready for strengthening. Remember, this can take anywhere from a few days to a few months depending on the level of complexity of the issue, how many different structures are affected and how long someone has suffered. Don't rush it. If you try to start the strengthening exercises too soon, you will flare up your tendon. If that happens, you will then have to wait until it settles back down again which will take longer to ultimately heal.

This is where the magic happens

This is my favorite phase of the whole program, as this is where the magic happens, and the tendon heals. I love empowering people to get to and through this phase because I see such a change in their demeanor and outlook once they realize they are in control of their symptoms and their recovery. Most people are surprised to learn that there is just one strengthening exercise they need to do to heal their tendon. Maybe it's because they've been given lists of dozens of exercises in the past. However, when you cut away all the "fluff", there is only one exercise that heals the tendon.

Once you are doing the strengthening exercise, you will become pain free, if you haven't already. You will need to slowly build up the weight as you get comfortable with the exercise and get stronger. Most clients who want to get back to low intensity activities will build up to using between 5- and 8-pound (2 to 3.5kg) dumbbells. Clients who want to return to mid-level intensity activities will build to between 8- and 12-pound (3.5 to 5.5kg) dumbbells. Clients who want to return to high intensity activities such as tennis or golf will build to between 12-to-15-pound (5.5 to 7kg) dumbbells.

As with the previous chapters, we'll cover the strengthening exercise you need to heal your tendon first. If you've been feeling symptoms for less than 3 months, you may just need the first exercise. If you've been feeling it for longer, you'll need the rest.

The Comprehensive Elbow Pain Relief Program contains 15 specific strengthening exercises that focus on the entire kinetic chain from the core to the fingers and everything in between. If you have a chronic condition and are aiming to completely resolve your tennis elbow once and for all, you not only need to regain the strength in the weak muscles around the elbow but also address any weaknesses around the shoulder and spine too.

1. Heavy load eccentric training

I can actually remember the day that I heard about this ground-breaking research that came out of Sweden. One of the senior physios (physical therapists) came racing into the department where I was working, clutching this article and stating that it was going to change everything. She was indeed correct. (Jo Gibson, that was you!) The contents of this article enabled me to treat Achilles tendinopathies incredibly successfully. One patient's Achilles was so bad it looked like there was a small plum on the tendon. However, the patient rehabbed it so well that when I bumped into him 6 months later, neither of us could remember which side had been affected and you couldn't tell by looking at it!

Anyway, I digress. Back to the groundbreaking research from Sweden. Alfredson et al (1998) had tested a novel way of strengthening on a group of runners who had Achilles tendinopathy and couldn't run. *"After the 12-week training period, all 15 patients were back at their preinjury levels with full running activity. There was a significant decrease in pain during activity, and the calf muscle strength on the injured side had increased significantly and did not differ significantly from that of the non injured side. A comparison group of 15 recreational athletes with the same diagnosis and a long duration of symptoms had been treated conventionally, i.e. rest, nonsteroidal anti-inflammatory drugs, changes of shoes or orthoses, physical therapy, and in all cases also with ordinary training programs. In no case was the conventional treatment successful, and all patients were ultimately treated surgically. Our treatment model with heavy-load eccentric calf muscle training has a very good short-term effect on athletes in their early forties."*

Wow! Just wow! 100% success rate! Sounds too good to be true, doesn't it? And if we really pick it apart, there were ONLY 15 runners studied with the intervention. Although, I'm sure they were happy to be in the intervention group and back to running in 12 weeks, rather than surgery like the control group did. And if it works SO well, why doesn't everyone use it? This is a question I often ask myself! Indeed, the authors even questioned themselves. So, Fahlstrom et al (2003) repeated the study, but this time on 101 tendons. They found the same results. *"During the 12-week study, recreational athletes with mid-tendon tendinopathy found their pain decreased from 7/10 to 1/10 and they all got back to running."*

Heavy load eccentric exercise for tennis elbow

This is where the magic happens. There's a very specific way of doing the exercise that will heal your tendon. There is a portion of the movement that is helpful. There's a portion of the movement that is detrimental. This is crucial to get right from the outset. Set yourself up for success with this exercise.

Use the edge of a table or desk to support your arm. Move your chair, so you've likely got one leg on either side of the table leg and the edge of the table is lined up with the center of your body. Rest your affected arm on the table with your hand over the edge and your palm down towards the floor. If the edge of the table is sharp you can put a towel on it to protect the underneath part of your forearm and wrist. You need to be close to the table and have your arm as close to your body as possible.

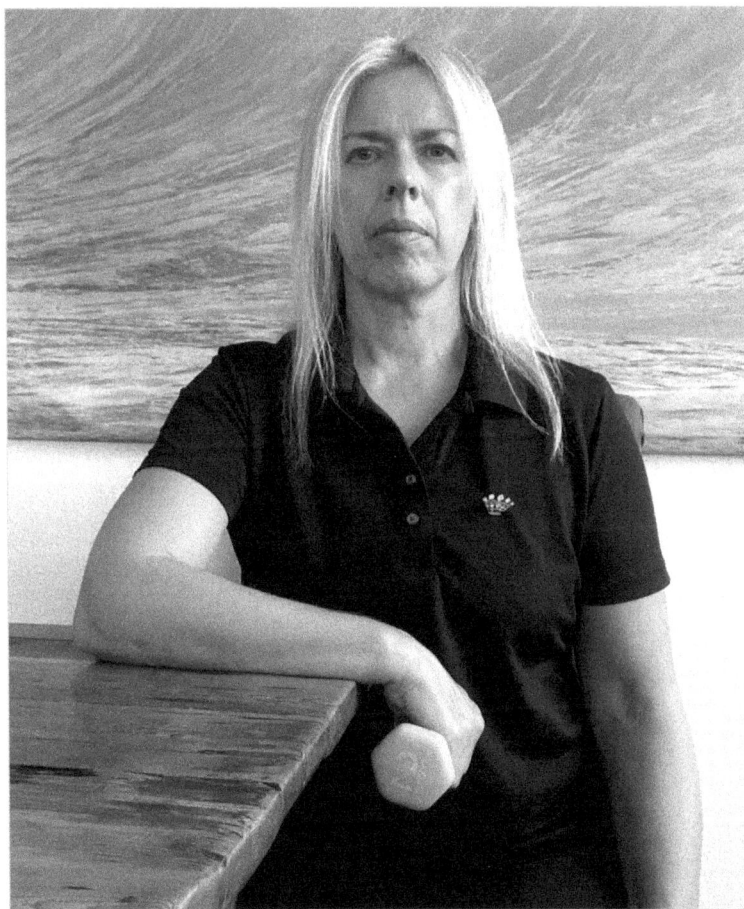

Gently hold a small dumbbell in your hand, not a death grip - that switches on all of the muscles, and will pull on the tendon. Use a maximum of 3 pounds (1.5kg) initially. The longer you have felt symptoms, the lighter the weight you need to start with. Some people may need to start with no weight at all. Allow your hand to lower down with gravity.

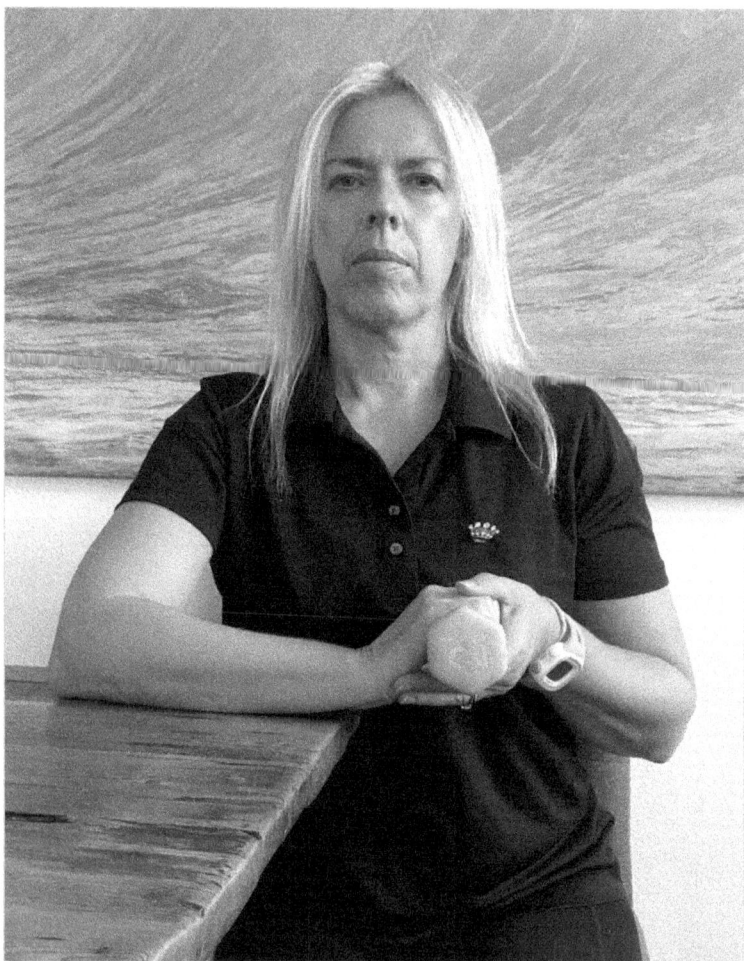

Use the other hand to pick it up because if you were to lift it using the muscles, that would irritate the tendon. So use the other hand to lift it and then let go to take the strain at the very top of the movement. Then lower it down. The lowering with control strengthens and lengthens the muscle and heals the tendon. Bring the other hand underneath again, to pick the weight back up and then lower it down with control again. This is the sequence; pick up with the unaffected hand, lower down using the affected side by itself.

When doing this, you want to be very mindful of what you are feeling in your elbow and forearm. If it's feeling easy, do 15 reps and then stop and stretch. You're always going to do the forearm stretch you learned in the previous chapter, straight after each set of strengthening exercises because the muscle tension goes up with strengthening exercises. If the muscle tension gets high enough, it will pull on the tendon. So use the forearm stretch, for 30 seconds after each set to bring the muscle tension back down.

If 15 repetitions feel okay to start with, try 3 sets; do another set of 15, then stretch again, and then do a third set of 15 reps and then stretch. If you're feeling any irritation with this keep the number of reps lower. You could start with 10 or even less. Let yourself be comfortable.

Do this twice a day. Do it in the morning and do it in the afternoon or evening. Your ultimate goal with this exercise is that you do 3 sets of 15 reps twice a day. That would be 15 reps and then stretch, 15 reps and stretch, 15 reps and stretch in the morning. 15 reps and stretch, 15 reps and stretch, 15 reps and stretch in the afternoon or evening. That's 90 repetitions every day of a movement that you've not done before.

The reason you need to start conservatively with this is that you don't want to irritate anything. Overuse or the hypersensitized nervous system can lead to fast irritation if you are not in the correct position or you do too much, too soon. If you start doing a lot of these motions and you don't build up slowly and gradually, you're just going to irritate your thumb or some of the other tendons around the wrist and hand. Once you get comfortable doing this with the light weight (or without any weight) and you get up to 3 sets of 15, twice a day, those numbers never change. The only thing that will change is that the weight will get heavier.

You are going to do these exercises for at least 12 months. Make a note of today's date here. This is the day that you're starting these exercises:

DATE:

Now, make a note of the date in 12 months time:

DATE:

As you begin to strengthen, you will start to notice a big difference in how your elbow is feeling. It takes 6 weeks of doing an exercise to build up strength. Having said that, most people start to feel better after about 2 to 3 weeks. It is not because they're stronger because truly they're not. In reality, the muscles are working better so they start feeling better.

When to increase the weight

Start increasing the weight when it feels too easy. Get up to 3 sets of 15 reps, twice a day with no weight. Once that's comfortable, start adding weight. Start with 1 or 2 pounds (0.5-1 kg). Do 3 sets of 15, twice a day. When you get to the point where you feel this is easy, maybe you could do 3 sets of 20, then it's not heavy enough and you need to increase the weight. Build up sequentially, pound by pound (half kilo by half kilo) ideally. If you try a big jump, sometimes it can irritate the tendon.

On my website, there's an example of adjustable dumbbells that take you from 2.5 pounds to 11 pounds (1kg to 5kg). Generally speaking, everybody needs to get up to at least 5 pounds (2.25kg). At that point, most people are comfortable doing day to day activities around the house. I've had clients reach 8 pounds (3.75kg) and be fine to play pickleball or go kayaking. If you want to get back to playing tennis or golf, you are more likely to need to get up to 12 pounds plus (5.5kg). You might need to get up to 15 pounds (7kg). It's very individual. If you're still feeling symptoms when you're picking something up, you're not heavy enough yet and you need to continue to get heavier until you reach the point when you are symptom-free and you're able to do everything you want to do. Do these exercises for at least 12 months.

Eccentric vs concentric loading

Concentric muscle activation shortens the muscle. Think of a bicep curl - as you bend your elbow taking your hand closer to your shoulder, the biceps muscle shortens. Eccentric muscle activation lowers the weight back down under control. When doing a bicep curl, you're holding the weight by your shoulder and slowly allowing your elbow to straighten down. This part of the movement is an eccentric muscle contraction of the biceps. The biceps muscle is lengthening to control the weight back down. This is eccentric muscle activation in action.

Researchers have wondered about the specific type of loading (eccentric) they were doing to the tendon in the previous successful studies and compared it with more "regular" loading (concentric). Think about the usual wrist curl exercises you have probably done before. THINK about them, but don't do them! Here's why: Mafi et al (2001) found *"the results showed that after the eccentric training regimen 82% of the patients were satisfied and had resumed their previous activity level (before injury), compared to 36% of the patients who were treated with the concentric training regimen."*

Peterson et al (2014) found *"eccentric graded exercise reduced pain and increased muscle strength in chronic tennis elbow more effectively than concentric graded exercise."*

My theory is that the concentric version pulls on the tendon as it shortens. This pulling irritates the tendon and therefore, it struggles to heal. The eccentric version lengthens the muscle as it's loading the tendon and the tendon likes this type of load. Some of my patients have described the eccentric exercises as feeling "soothing". This is perhaps a good time to remind you that the exercises should feel comfortable. "No pain, no gain" has no place here.

So having learned this strategy in 1998 and used it incredibly successfully on Achilles tendinopathy patients in the early to mid 2000s, I used the principles to come up with the exercise that ultimately healed Buddy. There has been some trial and error over the years regarding the best position to be in when you do the exercises and the best resistance to use, but I'll guide you through so you don't make the same mistakes I've made in the past.

How often should you do the eccentric exercises? Every single day, no days off. "But Emma, shouldn't you have a rest day?" Not when you are rehabbing your tendon. Take off your fitness hat and put on your rehab hat. Knobloch (2007) found *"daily eccentric training for Achilles tendinopathy is a safe and easy measure, with beneficial effects on the microcirculatory tendon levels without any evident adverse effects.*" We apply this principle to the common extensor tendon of the elbow.

What about isometrics?

Isometric describes a muscle contraction without moving – think holding a weight out in front of you without moving. The muscles may have to work hard, but your body isn't moving. Isotonic describes muscle activity with movement.

It's worth mentioning another form of muscle action here too. It has been reported that isometric (static) contractions can be helpful in the early stages of tendon rehabilitation. The response to isometric exercise is variable both within and across tendinopathy populations. However, Stasinopoulos (2022) stated that *"based on the literature, isometric exercise does not appear to be superior to isotonic exercise in the rehabilitation of chronic tendinopathy."*

Coombes et al (2016) found *"individuals with lateral epicondylalgia demonstrated increased pain intensity after an acute bout of isometric exercise."* For these reasons, I rarely utilize isometric exercises. I have tried them with a couple of patients who were struggling to complete the eccentric exercises but found them to be of limited effectiveness. Indeed, if radial tunnel syndrome is causing part of the symptoms, then isometric exercises can cause an increase in symptoms.

What does the research show?

Cook et al (2016) stated that *"exercise and load management are fundamental to [the] management [of tendon pathology]."*

Ohberg et al (2004) showed a *"localized decrease in tendon thickness and a normalized tendon structure in patients with chronic Achilles tendinosis after treatment with eccentric training."*

Vicenzino (2003) states *"The primary physical impairment in lateral epicondylalgia is a deficit in grip strength predominantly due to pain and its consequences on motor function* (how you can use your arm). *Hence the mainstay of successful management of this condition is therapeutic exercise, provided it is not pain provocative."* This is worth repeating yet again: providing it doesn't hurt!

Hoogvliet et al (2013) showed that *"strength training decreases symptoms in lateral epicondylitis."* Indeed, I often hear this from my clients. One gentleman told me, "My elbow felt a little sore when I started the first set, but the second and third sets really felt soothing. It doesn't make sense to me." It makes PERFECT sense; tendons LOVE load, and they especially love the specific eccentric load that heals them and soothes them in the process.

Ortega-Castillo et al (2016) found that *"pain decreased significantly with eccentric exercise."* Then Ortega-Castillo et al (2022) stated *"evidence that supported progressive exercise with eccentric components in adding a significant effect on pain and function."*

Yoon et al (2021) found *"eccentric exercise can improve pain and muscle strength in patients with lateral elbow tendinopathy."*

How long do you need to do the exercises for?

You know you need to do daily eccentric exercises to heal your tendon, but how long do you need to do them for? Chen et al (2021) found *"a treatment program using eccentric strengthening of **adequate intensity and duration** seemed to be most effective for treating lateral elbow tendinopathy."* But what is the adequate intensity and duration? This is where my 15 years of experience comes in. You have to get heavy to heal the tendon. While you start the exercises with weenie weights to allow the tissues to increase their tolerance to the stresses and strains we're putting through them, you cannot HEAL with weenie weights!

I've helped many clients who had rehabbed their elbows well but just couldn't get back on court. Every time they tried to play, their elbows hurt. When I asked them how heavy they were doing their eccentrics, they told me 2–3 pounds (1 kg). This is nowhere near heavy enough to be able to tolerate hitting a tennis ball.

In my experience, the following zones apply:

- Between 5-8# (2.25-3.5kg) most people are comfortable doing normal day-to-day activities
- Between 8-12# (3.5kg-5.5kg) most people are comfortable doing moderate-intensity activities
- But to do high-intensity activities like tennis, golf, weightlifting, playing the drums etc, you need to be 12#+ (5.5kg+)

Now, even though you know you've got to get heavy with the weights, (the protocol is called HEAVY load eccentric exercises after all), you shouldn't get too heavy too quickly. Slowly build up your weight, this allows the tissues to increase their tolerance to what you are asking them to do. Jump up in weight too quickly and you could flare your symptoms up. Also getting TOO heavy for your body can also cause issues. Makes sense really doesn't it?

To address the question of how long to do the exercises: It was general opinion that tendons healed in 12 weeks.[35] Indeed, if you think back to the groundbreaking research done on Achilles tendons, they followed the program for 12 weeks. Back when I was working with Buddy and all the tennis elbow sufferers that swiftly followed him, the advice was to do the heavy load eccentric exercises for 12 weeks. And that works to get you to the pain-free point. However, Li et al (2021) found that *"the remodeling phase of tendon healing starts 1–2 months after injury and spans more than 1 year. Maybe even up to two years in some individuals."* So, now the recommendation is to do the eccentrics for **at least 12 months**.[36]

2. Central sensitization

Heales et al (2014) found *"deficits in sensory and motor systems present bilaterally in unilateral tendinopathy. This implies potential central nervous system involvement. This indicates that rehabilitation should consider the contralateral side of patients."* So, it's important to do many of the exercises on both sides. If you've been feeling symptoms for longer than 3 months, this is crucial to address and is often the limiting factor for people who have "failed" therapy or other treatments previously. This can be addressed by a knowledgeable practitioner.

3. TNT – This will blow your mind

Rio et al, 2016 found:

- Tendinopathy may be associated with changes in motor control; these changes may be bilateral and persistent despite rehabilitation.

- Current rehabilitation may not adequately address motor control issues as self-paced strength training (the mainstay of the treatment) does not alter corticospinal drive to the muscle—this may contribute to recalcitrance and recurrence of tendinopathy.

- Tendon neuroplastic training (TNT) proposes a concept of strength-based loading that is an important stimulus for tendon and muscle, but with strategies known to optimize neuroplasticity of the motor cortex and drive to the muscle.

So what does that actually mean?

Your tennis elbow may lead to your muscles not working quite as well as they used to. This has nothing to do with weakness. It's all to do with how well the muscles switch on and work when you're doing an activity. This doesn't only affect your painful side, it can affect BOTH arms. The heavy eccentric loading will reduce pain, increase strength and allow you to return to doing all the activities you love. However, your muscles may not be working as well as they used to before the injury.

Welsh (2018) suggests that *"the central nervous system may play a role in chronic tendinopathies. It is possible that TNT may address the central nervous system component of chronic/recurrent tendinopathy that is not addressed by traditional passive therapies. TNT combines strength training with an externally paced audio or visual cue. Patients perform a strength training task that loads the affected tendon. Rather than a self-paced maneuver, the patient matches the speed of the exercise to the audio and/or visual cue provided by a metronome. Retraining the brain to decrease pain with external pacing is easy to implement and may prove to become a valuable addition to traditional tendon rehabilitation loading protocols."*

In a nutshell, use a metronome while doing your eccentric exercises and your muscles will recover better. (I told you this would blow your mind!) I advise you to set the metronome (or app on your phone) to 60 beats a minute. Lift up for the first beat, then lower down for 3 beats. It is essential that you can see and hear the metronome to get the effect of TNT. If you just count in your head, you are doing yourself a disservice and your muscles will likely not recover as well as they could have done.

4. The best core exercise... ever

There is a simple and effective exercise that most people can do to start engaging the core muscles correctly. It's pelvic floor exercises aka Kegels. The Transversus Abdominis (core muscle) and pelvic floor muscles work together as they are so internal. You can use the pelvic floor muscles to initiate a true core contraction. This is a very different feeling to just pulling your stomach in, as it's very internal. You switch on transversus abdominis, however it takes some practice.

For most people, these muscles are not doing what they need to do. You need to get them switched back on because your core should be activated at a low level for you all day long. Transversus abdominis is an endurance muscle or a marathon muscle, it's not a sprint muscle. For example, think about working a fast twitch or sprint muscle like your biceps. If you were to do bicep curls, the muscle would switch on, switch off, switch on, switch off, as you raised your hand up and down. Transversus abdominis doesn't work like that. Transversus abdominis should be switched on at a low level of contraction, and then kept on. It's more about endurance than speed.

Basically, because the transversus abdominis muscle is so internal, it works in conjunction with the pelvic floor muscles. Start practicing these exercises lying down because there's no weight going through your body and particularly your spine, in a lying down position. The spine is also in a nice supported neutral posture position. Remember the position you started the knee rolling exercise in? That's how you're going to start the core exercises too.

Put your hands on your tummy. One hand below your belly button and one hand on your tummy above your belly button.

Don't push or press, you're just going to feel what the abdominal muscles are doing. Now, try and suck in your lower tummy. It's like sucking in your gut. What happens with most people is that all the abs work together, because when your brain sends the message down to your stomach to say, "Switch on," all of the abdominals want to help. So, by consciously thinking about sucking your tummy in, you likely struggle to get a pure core contraction because everything switches on.

A different way to think about this is by using a pelvic floor contraction. An easy way to do this is by using Kegels. The pelvic floor muscles and the deep core muscle work together. You can do a pelvic floor contraction and get a sneaky switch on of transversus abdominis as well. Essentially, you're just going to imagine you're in the restroom, urinating, and stop the flow. Use the muscles that you'd use to stop peeing. Use those muscles to get a core contraction and start engaging transversus abdominis correctly.

Keep breathing normally. You shouldn't be holding your breath. You want to switch the muscles on and keep them on but keep breathing. Hold the muscle contraction for about 10 seconds, then release it. Switch on again. Keep breathing normally. Hold for 10 seconds. Try to do 10 repetitions at a time and try to do that every hour throughout the day. Yes, you need to be practicing it little and often. The key with transversus abdominis is it should be switched on for you all day long, and for most people, it's not. Add in back pain, pregnancies or abdominal surgeries over the years, and transversus abdominis is most likely switched off.

Check out a series of videos showing how you can start getting these muscles switched on in the book bonuses:

http://bit.ly/TE-bookbonuses

It is a good idea to get some guidance with regards to this if you are not sure if you are doing it correctly. You should not feel any pain or discomfort as you do any of these exercises. If you do, something's not right. You could be in a poor position or the muscles are not switching on correctly. If you're feeling discomfort, something is not okay, so check in with an experienced physical therapist.

6. Upper quadrant strengthening

If you've suffered for longer that 3 months, you may also need to strengthen your:

- Neck
- Shoulder blade
- Rotator cuff

If you have several tendons affected or you want to return to a rotational activity like tennis or golf, you may also need to strengthen your:

- Biceps
- Triceps
- Pronators
- Supinators

Depending on your needs these may need to be eccentrically focused. An experienced localized practitioner can customize your plan for you.

Day et al (2015) found *"when compared to a matched comparison group, there were impairments of scapular musculature strength and endurance in patients with lateral epicondylalgia, suggesting that the scapular musculature should be assessed and potentially treated in this population. Cause and effect cannot be established, as the weakness of the scapular musculature could be a result of lateral epicondylalgia."* Yes, absolutely true. But also irrelevant to the patient. There's a weakness that's associated with your issue in some way. It needs addressing.

Sethi et al (2018) found that *"scapular muscle strengthening should be used along with the conventional physiotherapy in individuals with chronic lateral epicondylalgia to improve pain, pain free grip strength, functional outcome, muscle strength, scapular position and muscle activity."*

Ucurum et al (2019) found *"upper extremity muscle strength, grip strength, and scapular position are affected in patients with lateral epicondylalgia. In addition to the elbow, focusing on the upper segments is essential in the management of lateral epicondylalgia."*

This is why the Comprehensive Elbow Pain Relief Program focuses on strengthening these elements and it also addresses the core and neck too. If your practitioner is only focusing on your elbow, it's time to find a new practitioner!

6. Regain proprioception

Proprioception is the ability to know where your body is in space, without looking at it. I know it sounds a bit odd, but it's a crucial element in recovery and prevention of injury. You're doing all this great work at healing the injury you've been dealing with. Regaining proprioception will help to fully heal it AND prevent other injuries in the future!

Taking weight through your arm improves proprioception. The heavy load eccentric exercises will help this to a degree, as will weight-bearing exercises that you'll likely need as you strengthen your shoulder. An experienced local practitioner can help you with this.

Juul-Kristensen (2008) found *"proprioception seems to be poorer in elbows with lateral epicondylitis than in the controls' elbows. This needs to be taken into consideration in the management of lateral epicondylitis."*

Interestingly, Stasinopoulos (2019) stated *"therapists ignore reduced proprioception in the management of lateral elbow tendinopathy. Reduced proprioception delays the healing process."* Stasinopoulos (2022) concluded, *"if physiotherapists use modalities to improve proprioception, the results will be effective sooner."*

Schiffke-Juhász et al (2021) found that *"12-week proprioceptive training improves pain, quality of life, grip strength and vibration sensation in patients with painful lateral epicondylitis."*

Why this is crucial for your recovery

Do you have to do these exercises for the rest of your life? We all should be. It's when people don't do the things that they should, that they get pain and problems developing. We should move our bodies as they were designed to move.

In people with tennis elbow, widespread strength deficits, including weakness of the shoulder, forearm, and wrist muscles, may exist. Heales et al (2021) reported *"some of these weaknesses appear on both the affected and the unaffected sides in people with tennis elbow. A physical therapist can help strengthen these areas".* The Comprehensive Elbow Pain Relief Program addresses these deficits but that is beyond the scope of this book.

Activity-specific progressions

This is when you can start increasing the intensity of your activity-specific movements. It's time to break out the racket or the club for example. But just start by testing out the super slow movements you were doing in phase 2. Practice a super slow serve motion. Try a golf swing. You are not hitting a ball to start with. Remember, that you still need to keep yourself 100% comfortable. It's never the time to push into pain. However, if you find you can comfortably complete all the movements you would do in your sport, in slo-mo, then you can start to increase the speed until you reach normal motion. Once you can complete full-speed movements, you can add a light ball. Think wiffle ball. Then you can progress to a light children's ball and finally a regular ball. Build up your tolerance.

Once you have been pain-free for a full week, doing all your normal daily activities, picking up your coffee cup or a bottle of water, lifting groceries or your laptop, turning a door handle or taking the lid off a jar, everything. Then, and only then, can you progress to Phase 4, regaining endurance, function and everything you want to be doing with no restrictions. This is an incredibly strict timeline, as if you try to progress too soon, you will flare up the tendon. That means that if you have gone for 6 days pain-free but then feel a little discomfort on day 7, you have to start counting your week again . Don't try to rush this part, you've come so far, don't jeopardize your progress . Be truly honest with yourself .

Find a checklist later in the book and download it here:

http://bit.ly/TE-bookbonuses

Let's continue to phase 4.

TENNIS ELBOW
QUEEN

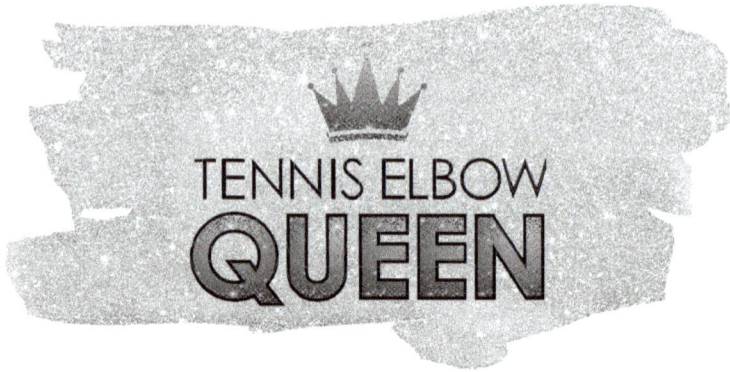

" My tennis elbow hadn't got any better with 6 months of trying YouTube videos and using the Theraband flexbar. Within a week of following Emma's advice, my elbow was feeling significantly better and I have been able to return to playing golf after just 8 weeks. "

M 39

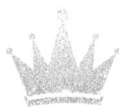

CHAPTER 10

Phase 4
Regaining Endurance and Function

Phase 4 Goals

- Regain endurance and function
- Begin return to high-intensity activities once you have been completely pain-free for a week doing all your normal activities
- Return to high-intensity activities
- Return to sport – no restrictions
- Nerve mobilizations (if needed)

Once you get established with the strengthening exercises, you will become pain-free and that's when you can start to think about getting back to all the activities you want to do. To progress from Phase Three, strengthening, into Phase Four, building endurance and regaining function, you must have been completely pain-free for a whole week doing all your normal activities. That means no twinge, no ache, no shadow of something, no difference to the unaffected side at all. Once you reach that point, you are ready to regain your more intensive activities and you can do this gradually and methodically, by only adding in one new exercise at a time, if you are returning to the gym or weight-lifting or gradually increasing the amount you play if you're returning to playing a musical instrument or a sport.

It's a slow and steady process to allow the tissues to acclimate to the new stresses and strains you are putting through them. I liken this process to that of a marathon runner. If you are brand new to marathon running, you don't get up one day and run 26.2 miles. You spend 6 months training and building up your stamina. You are essentially training the tissues of your body to tolerate the intensity of running 26 miles. You will use the same principle to get yourself safely and comfortably back to your activities. It does require some patience, but you know that it takes 12 months for the tendon to fully resolve anyway, so there's no rush.

1. Regain endurance

You've been building strength by doing the heavy load eccentric exercises; three sets of 15, twice a day. You've been doing your cardio exercise, to keep your fitness up. You've been doing visualization so you've kept the neural pathways strong so you can get back to doing the things that you want to do.

Whatever activity you want to get back to doing, you're going to build yourself up a little bit at a time, so that the tissues can tolerate it. If you do it that way, there is little chance of irritating anything.

2. Regain function

Let's talk about function. You should have been able to get back to doing pretty much everything classified as activities of daily living. Whatever you do during the day, you should be doing completely fine, and have no issues. Making your coffee in the morning, being able to pick up your cup, reaching into the fridge to grab the gallon of milk, picking up groceries and putting them into the trunk of your car. You should be able to mop a floor or do the vacuuming.

There might be some things that you're feeling a little cautious about doing and that's okay. You may have developed tennis elbow by laying a patio in the backyard and you think to yourself, maybe I'm not going to do that anymore. Well, you're going to be healed to such a point that you're going to be able to do whatever you want to do. You are going to be able to lift heavy stones or go and trim trees or use the shears when you're out in the backyard, or painting the fence. It's quite normal to feel apprehension about some of these movements, particularly if it's something out of the ordinary like painting a fence or laying a patio. Maybe something like this has flared your elbow up in the past. You'll be able to do whatever you want to do, completely pain-free, with no restrictions. You shouldn't ever have to think, I can't do that because of my elbow or I mustn't do that because of my elbow. The only time you could potentially flare it is if you go back to these things too fast or if you go back too soon.

3. How long does each phase take?

This is a great question that I can answer with "How long is a piece of string?" Everybody is different, but know that these are the phases that you have to go through. If you try to skip a phase, you're not going to heal. The symptoms will come back.

Some people can get through phase 1 and phase 2 in a couple of weeks, be pain-free, have normal muscle tension, and be ready for the strengthening phase. Other clients spend longer in phases 1 and 2, particularly if they have been feeling the symptoms for a longer time, or have more structures involved, such as the neck and shoulder as well as the elbow. This can also be the case with clients who experience nerve symptoms, as this can lengthen the time needed in the first two phases.

Everybody needs to do the heavy load eccentric exercises for at least 12 months. But what happens then? Some clients would say, "I am never stopping these exercises because I feel good and I don't want the pain to ever come back." Some clients would wean down to do the exercises every other day, and that would keep them ticking over. Some clients would do them once a week, just to keep topped up, others would be able to wean down completely and never have to do the exercises again.

Generally, the length of time you have had tennis elbow symptoms before you start doing the right things is the length of time it's going to take for it to get better. So, if you've been suffering for 3 months, it can settle down in 3 months as long as you do the correct things. However, if you've had this for seven years, thankfully, it won't take seven years to settle down, and you will probably be better in around seven months. Now I know that still sounds like a long time, but it's not seven years. Most people can be better in 12 months, even if you've had it for three years, seven years or 30 years.

Most chronic tennis elbow sufferers are better within six or seven months. Sometimes a little bit longer if it's a more complex case with multiple tissues involved. But some people see a difference almost immediately. Everybody is different and it depends on where you are on your journey.

When you look at the phases of healing:

- Phase 1 settling the symptoms down, which generally, takes a week or so to integrate the strategies.
- Phase 2 normalizes the soft tissues. Again, looking at a week or so within that phase.
- Phase 3 is strengthening. You are going to be doing your strengthening exercises for at least 12 months.
- Phase 4 builds back your endurance and your function; getting you back in the gym, getting you back doing anything and everything. You need normal stresses and strains going through the tissues for good healing and normal stresses and strains are going to the gym, playing your musical instrument, doing housework, and doing yard work. It's all the activities that you do.

4. Nerve mobilizations

This is the phase in which specific nerve mobilizations are added, if not before. This is a very individual issue and one that I currently guide clients through on a personal basis. The reason for this is that it is extremely easy to flare nerves up, by doing the wrong movement at the wrong time or even for the wrong amount of time. If you have nerve symptoms, get guidance from a specialist physical therapist on how best to resolve your specific nerve issues.

Basson et al (2020) found *"The UCNM [usual care plus nerve mobilization] group had significantly less pain at 6-month follow-up and a lower mean pain rating at 12-month follow-up."*

Ellis et al (2022) stated *"Whilst the early use of neurodynamics was centered within a mechanical paradigm, research into the working mechanisms of tensioning techniques revealed neuroimmune, neurophysiological, and neurochemical effects. In-vitro and ex-vivo research confirms that tensile loading is required for mechanical adaptation of healthy and healing neurons and nerves. Moreover, elimination of tensile load can have detrimental effects on the nervous system. Beneficial effects of tensile loading and tensioning techniques, contributing to restored homeostasis at the entrapment site, dorsal root ganglia and spinal cord, include neuronal cell differentiation, neurite outgrowth and orientation, increased endogenous opioid receptors, reduced fibrosis and intraneural scar formation, improved nerve regeneration and remyelination, increased muscle power and locomotion, less mechanical and thermal hyperalgesia and allodynia, and improved conditioned pain modulation. However, animal and cellular models also show that 'excessive' tensile forces have negative effects on the nervous system. Although robust and designed to withstand mechanical load, the nervous system is equally a delicate system. Mechanical loads that can be easily handled by a healthy nervous system, may be sufficient to aggravate clinical symptoms in patients."*

Nuñez de Arenas-Arroyo et al (2022) found that *"neurodynamic techniques improved intraneural edema dispersion."*

Last thoughts

Make sure that you take your time with everything. Look at it more like marathon training rather than sprint training. It is over a longer time because the research shows that if you stop doing the exercises too soon, there's a potential that the tendon may not be completely healed, and the symptoms could return

Keep doing the exercises for at least 12 months and all the other elements that feel good. If you want to keep doing heat, keep doing heat. Keep doing cardio exercise, meditation, progressive relaxation, visualization, and watching your posture. All of these different elements are focused on healing your tennis elbow. But they're good for general health and wellbeing too. When you get enough sleep and get good nutrition, you feel better. We all know that. So look at this now as you've set up some great habits to follow. You've changed your lifestyle. You've set up some outstanding routines. Maybe you're doing progressive relaxation every night. Keep it up, it's going to be helpful. All of these strategies were focused on resolving tennis elbow but they are all immensely helpful for health and wellbeing as well. So keep going. You've done fantastically well.

So there you have it. Your plan for healing your tennis elbow. If you have any questions, don't hesitate to reach out to:

Emma@TennisElbowQueen.com

You can find my website at www.TennisElbowQueen.com

Find me on social media at:

Facebook:
https://www.facebook.com/TennisElbowQueenPT

Instagram:
https://www.instagram.com/tenniselbowqueen/

YouTube:
https://www.youtube.com/c/
EmmaGreenTennisElbowQueen

TENNIS ELBOW QUEEN

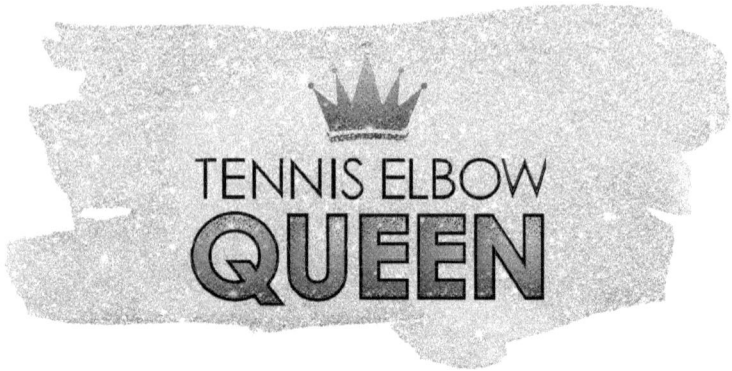

66 Emma gets a gold star for giving me the right advice. The Dr was so impressed by how much I'd Improved since my last appointment. I never thought I would get back to playing hockey again, but I was back playing within 3 months of following Emma's advice. I had no idea this would work. 99

KH 46

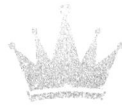

Next Steps

30-Day Guide

First things first, start to implement everything you've learned in this book. You'll find a handy 30-day plan in the next section. This will give you guidance and structure to implement everything you've learned, without leaving anything out, so that you can start to feel better. Don't forget to grab the extra bonuses too:

http://bit.ly/TE-bookbonuses

Facebook group

Come and join the Elbow Pain Relief Facebook group. Buddy, my very first client, who you heard about earlier on, is in the group, and he is more than happy to talk to people about his experience resolving his elbow pain. The other clients who shared their success stories in this book, are in there too and want to give back. Please use it, it's a great resource and starting point. It's free to join. I'm in there a lot of the time, so if you have a question, you can catch me there. I love answering questions.

In the group, you'll find other people who are in the same situation as you and people who have been in the situation that you're in right now and are out the other side. It's one thing to hear it from me, but another to hear it from them. They were in your shoes. They can tell you what it was like to go through it and to live it and to have it behind them. I invite you to join my Facebook group here:

https://www.facebook.com/groups/tenniselbowrelief

Helpful hints emails

You can sign up for helpful hints emails in the Facebook group or by signing up for the book bonuses:

http://bit.ly/TE-bookbonuses

Online Comprehensive Elbow Pain Relief coaching program

This is for people who want more speciliazed guidance going through the healing process. Maybe you are feeling both elbows, or have golfer's elbow too, or feel your shoulder or neck. Maybe you just want to make absolutely sure that you're doing the right things at the right times. If so, you may benefit from specific guidance for your particular issues.

Learn more about the online Comprehensive Elbow Pain Relief Coaching Program here:

http://bit.ly/TE-bookbonuses

Your opportunity to work with Emma beyond this book

I really hope you've enjoyed reading this book as much as I have enjoyed writing it. You can probably tell I'm passionate about helping people. The reason I wrote this book was because I realized that I was saying the same things to every single client, and I thought, I should write this down and get it out there, so that more people can be helped. So, here we are, this is how it was created. One-on-one consultations limit the number of people that I can help. In a medium like this I can help people all over the world, anytime of the day or night, the information is available.

I work with a select number of clients, so if you absolutely want to work with me, one-on-one, there are possibilities for that. It might just be a one-off consultation, making sure that the program is right for your needs. Please email me to apply:

Emma@TennisElbowQueen.com

Let's get you back to doing everything you want to do as much as you want to do it. No restrictions. Don't live life in fear of pain. That's not living life. Let's not live life halfway, let's live life to the full. We're here for a very limited time. Let's enjoy it as much as we can. Thank you so much for joining me in this book.

TENNIS ELBOW
QUEEN

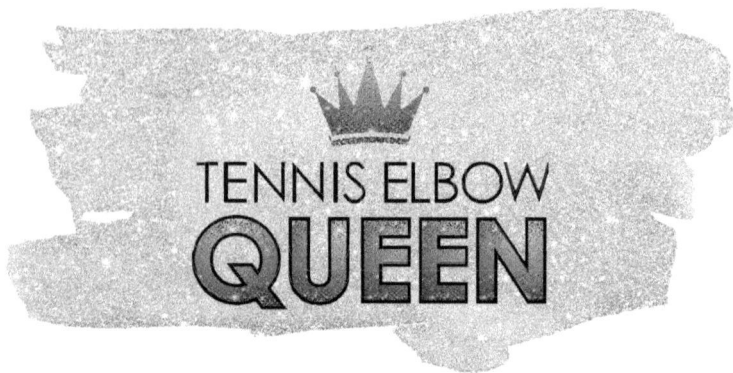

66I have just told my doctor that I feel the best I
have ever felt! This is working! Awesome!99

DB 29

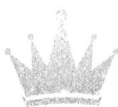

30-Day Guide

Y ou've learned a lot about tennis elbow and how to heal it. But now you need to start implementing. "But Emma, there are so many things to do, do I need to do all of them?"

Do you want to heal your tennis elbow? Every strategy is in for a reason. Trying to skip, will lead to longer healing time and potentially a worse outcome. Trust the process. This program has helped thousands of people all over the world. Take the knowledge you've learned and apply it. Don't hesitate to reach out if you need to. I can be reached here:

Emma@TennisElbowQueen.com

Before you start

It's really important to understand why you are doing certain things, otherwise you may find yourself skipping over certain strategies after a few days, forgetting to do them after a while or never doing them from the start. If you find yourself wondering why you are doing a particular thing, head back to the relevant chapter to refresh your memory as to why each section is needed.

The basic guidelines

These strategies need to be completed every single day with no days off. This is rehabilitation of your elbow, it's not fitness, so there are no rest days.

Try every single strategy. You may not need every one, but if you leave out something that you do need, you won't heal effectively. So, do it all to be on the safe side.

This book is not intended to diagnose any medical condition. See a doctor or other medical practitioner for that.

This book is not written for a specific person. I've included my knowledge of the many clients I have helped with their tennis elbows. I don't know you or your specific history. As such, you assume all risks associated with participating in a rehabilitation program, including getting clearance from your doctor prior to beginning any new exercise regime. You agree to hold harmless the author for any and all claims associated with participation in this rehabilitation program.

Worksheets

Scheduling the strategies into your day has proven to be a very effective way to complete the program. All the following resources are in the book bonuses:

http://bit.ly/TE-bookbonuses

Cardio Calendar

Here is my cardio calendar for you to use:

EMMA GREEN

1	2	3	4	5	6	7
1 minute! Great start!	2 minutes! Keep it up!	3 minutes	4 minutes	5 minutes	6 minutes	7 minutes 1 week done!
8	9	10	11	12	13	14
8 minutes	9 minutes	10 minutes Double figures!	11 minutes	12 minutes	13 minutes	14 minutes 2 weeks!!
15	16	17	18	19	20	21
15 minutes Halfway there!	16 minutes	17 minutes	18 minutes	19 minutes	20 minutes	21 minutes 3 weeks!!!
22	23	24	25	26	27	28
22 minutes	23 minutes	24 minutes	25 minutes	26 minutes	27 minutes	28 minutes 4 weeks!!!!
29	30	31				
29 minutes Almost to your goal!!!	30 minutes You did it!	30 minutes Whoop whoop!				

TENNIS ELBOW QUEEN

Cardio Challenge

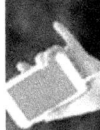

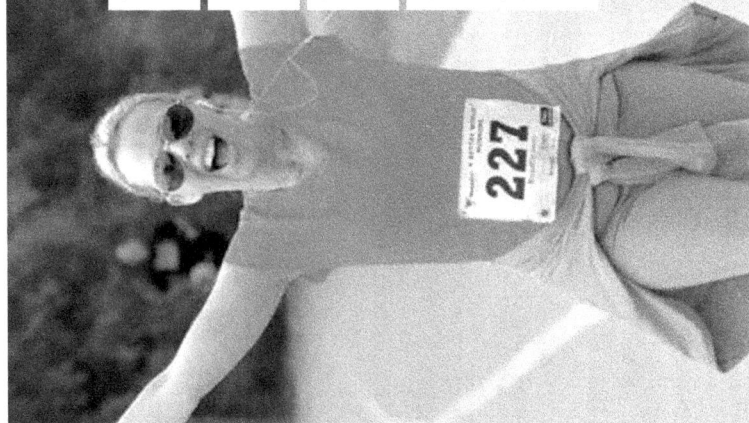

227

Tennis Elbow Checklist – Phases 1, 2 and 3

Daily List

- **Core exercises** Try to switch on the core muscles 10 times every hour through the day. Hold each rep for 10 seconds, but don't hold your breath.

- **Heat the elbow, neck, shoulder and forearm** for 10 minutes, at least 5 times per day.

- **Neck** Exercise 10 times, at least 3 times per day.

- **Trigger point** the upper traps and forearm muscles after the heat.

- **Soft tissue massage** on the forearm muscles after the heat.

- **Heavy load eccentrics** 3 sets of 15 twice a day, no days off.

- **Stretch** the upper traps and forearm (after each set of eccentrics), 30 second hold, at least 3 times per day.

- **Shoulder rolls** 10 reps at least 3 times per day.

- **Ice the elbow** for 3 days if you feel you have irritated it, then return to the heat.

- **Posture** Watch your posture, particularly when you are sitting. Set the timer on your phone for 20 minutes. When it goes off, stand up, sit down and resume a good posture.

- **Ergonomics** Use a wrist rest when you are typing and using the mouse.

- **Relative rest** Avoid any activities that make it hurt.

- **Brace** Use a tennis elbow strap if you cannot avoid a painful activity. But only use it when you really need it as it will weaken the muscles

- **Pills / potions / lotions** Take any pain medication, anti- inflammatories or muscle relaxers that have been prescribed to you by your doctor.

- **Sleep** Get 8 hours per night.
- **Nutrition** Eat a healthy diet (eg plant-based) ensuring protein at every meal and snack.
- **Hydration** 8 glasses of water per day.
- **Cardio** 30 minutes daily, ideally outside.
- **Progressive relaxation** Every night before going to sleep.
- **Meditation** 10-20 minutes daily.
- **Visualization daily** - start with a couple of minutes and build up. The more you do, the stronger the neural pathways stay.

TENNIS ELBOW QUEEN

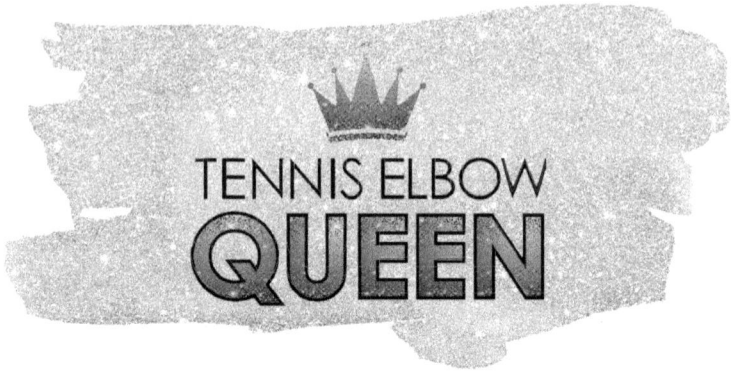

661 suffered with elbow pain for years! I was unable to play my violin or do any gardening. I was struggling using the mouse and couldn't go to the gym or lift anything. Less than 4 weeks into Emma's program and I can unload the dishwasher and make the bed with no pain. I played my violin for 6 hours yesterday with no pain and woke up feeling fine this morning.99

ML 58

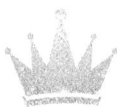

FAQs

How does the program help tennis elbow?

The Comprehensive Elbow Pain Relief Program is an all-encompassing, hurt to healed system that was developed in response to a need for a better way to treat and heal tennis elbow. It was extensively researched and evidence-based. It continues to evolve and change as new research is released, or more effective techniques are developed.

What makes the program different to other treatments out there?

This program addresses the nervous system, where most other treatments don't. It also developed into a logical system of treatment which is segmented into phases. Each phase builds on the previous phase to solidify your progress. Most general healthcare providers don't address the nervous system at all, let alone from day 1 and throughout the entire plan of care.

How do I join the program?

If you would like specific guidance on healing your elbow, the first step is to watch this webinar:

https://bit.ly/TEprogramLearnMore

Then you can book a call to discuss your suitability for the program and choose which option suits you best. Hope to see you on a call soon!

Questions to ask your healthcare provider

- How many tennis elbow clients do you see each week?
- What exercises will you start me with?
- How will you address the nervous system?
- How long will I need to do the exercises for?

You want to work with someone who treats multiple tennis elbow clients each week, that is someone who recognizes the involvement of other tissues. Someone who will give you advice regarding calming the nervous system down and who is aware of the research proving that tendons take at least 12 months to fully resolve. If you get these answers, jump right into their care. If you don't hear these answers, they may not be the specialist you are searching for and will struggle to give you the specialist knowledge and treatment that you require to fully resolve.

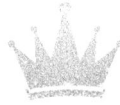

First Edition Reference List

1. Calfee, RP, Patel, A, DaSilva, MF, Akelman, E Management of lateral epicondylitis: current concepts *J. Am. Acad. Orthop. Surg.* 2008 1619–29

2. Cutts, S, Gangoo, S, Modi, N, Pasapula, C Tennis elbow: A Clinical review article *J. Orthop.* 2019 203–7

3. Kongsgaard M, Kovanen V, Aagaard P, et al .Corticosteroid injections, eccentric decline squat training and heavy slow resistance training in patellar tendinopathy . *Scand J Med Sci Sports.* 2009 790–802

4. Nichols AW . Complications associated with the use of corticosteroids in the treatment of athletic injuries . *Clin J Sport Med.* 2005;15(5):370–375

5. Brinks A, Koes BW, Volkers ACW, Verhaar JAN, Bierma-Zeinstra SMA Adverse effects of extra-articular cosrticosteroid injections: a systematic review . *BMC Musculoskelet Disord.* 2010 206

6. Coombes BK, Bisset L, Brooks P, Khan A, Vicenzino B. Effect of corticosteroid injection, physiotherapy, or both on clinical outcomes in patients with unilateral lateral epicondylalgia: a randomized controlled trial . *JAMA.* 2013 461–9

7. Connell D, Burke F, Coombes P et-al . Sonographic examination of lateral epicondylitis . *AJR Am J Roentgenol* . 2001 777–82

8. Martel MO, Finan PH, Dolman AJ, Sudramanian S, Edwards RR, Wasan AD, Jamison RN Self-reports of medication side effects and pain-related activity interference in patients with chronic pain: A longitudinal cohort study . *Pain.* 2015 1092–1110

9. Maffulli N, Moller HD, Evans CH Tendon healing: can it be optimised? *British Journal of Sports Medicine* 2002 315–316

10. Sharma P, Maffulli, N Biology of tendon injury: Healing, modeling and remodeling *Journal of musculoskeletal & neuronal interactions* 2005 181–90

11. Chanda ML, Alvin MD, Schnitzer TJ, Apkarian AV Pain characteristic differences between subacute and chronic back pain *J Pain* 2011 792–800

12. Öhberg L, Lorentzon R, Alfredson H Eccentric training in patients with chronic Achilles tendinosis: normalised tendon structure and decreased thickness at follow up *British Journal of Sports Medicine* 2004 8–11

13. Walz DM, Newman JS, Konin GP, Ross G Epicondylitis: Pathogenesis, Imaging, and Treatment *RadioGraphics* 2010 167–184

14. Booth PW Physiological and biochemical effects of immobilization on muscle . *Clinical Orthopedics and Related Research* 1987 15–20

15. Lindboe CP, Platou CS Effects of immobilization of short duration on muscle fibre size . *Clinical Physiology* 1984 183

16. Miles MP, Clarkson PM, Bean M, Ambach K, Mulroy J, Vincent K Muscle function at the wrist following 9 d of immobilization and suspension . *Med Sci Sports Exerc.* 1994 615–23

17. Clark BC, Manini TM, Hoffman RL, Russ DW Restoration of voluntary muscle strength after 3 weeks of cast immobilization is suppressed in women compared with men . *Arch Phys Med Rehabil.* 2009 178–80

18. Dingemanse R, Randsdorp M, Koes BW, Huisstede BM Evidence for the effectiveness of electrophysical modalities for treatment of medial and lateral epicondylitis: a systematic review . *Br J Sports Med.* 2014 957–65

19. Bisset L, Paungmali A, Vicenzino B, Beller E A systematic review and meta-analysis of clinical trials on physical interventions for lateral epicondylalgia . *Br J Sports Med.* 2005 411–22

20. Lai WC, Erickson BJ, Mlynarek RA, Wang D Chronic lateral epicondylitis: challenges and solutions . *Open Access J Sports Med* . 2018 243–251

21. Titchener AG, Fakis A, Tambe AA, Smith C, Hubbard RB, Clark DI Risk factors in lateral epicondylitis (tennis elbow): a case-control study . *Journal of Hand Therapy* 2012 159–64

22. Kim GK The Risk of Fluoroquinolone-induced Tendinopathy and Tendon Rupture: What Does The Clinician Need To Know? *J Clin Aesthet Dermatol* . 2010 49–54 .

23. Järvinen TA Neovascularisation in tendinopathy: from eradication to stabilisation? *British Journal of Sports Medicine* 2020 1–2

24. Grigg NL, Wearing SC, Smeathers JE Eccentric calf muscle exercise produces a greater acute reduction in Achilles tendon thickness than concentric exercise *British Journal of Sports Medicine* 2009 280–283

25. Yang S, Chang MC . Chronic Pain: Structural and Functional Changes in Brain Structures and Associated Negative Affective States . *Int J Mol Sci* . 2019 3130

26. Woolf CJ . Central sensitization: Implications for the diagnosis and treatment of pain . *Pain.* 2010;152(2 Suppl) S2–15

27. Gunn CC, Milbrandt WE . Tennis elbow and the cervical spine *Can Med Assoc J.* 1976 803–809

28. Smeets JS, Horstman AM, Vles GF, Emans PJ, Goessens JP, Gijsen AP, van Kranenburg JM, van Loon LJ Protein synthesis rates of muscle, tendon, ligament, cartilage, and bone tissue in vivo in humans *PLoS ONE* 2019 14

29. Seminowicz DA, Wideman TH, Naso L, Hatami-Khoroushahi Z, Fallatah S, Ware MA, Jarzem P, Bushnell MC, Shir Y, Ouellet JA, Stone LS Effective Treatment of Chronic Low Back Pain in Humans Reverses Abnormal Brain Anatomy and Function *Journal of Neuroscience* 2011 7540–7550

30. Young SN, Biologic effects of mindfulness meditation: growing insights into neurobiologic aspects of the prevention of depression *J Psychiatry Neurosci* . 2011 75–77

31. Ranganathan VK, Siemionow V, Liu JZ, Sahgal V, Yue GH From mental power to muscle power--gaining strength by using the mind . *Neuropsychologia.* 2004 944–56

32. Ayala Fde Baranda Andujar PS Effect of 3 different active stretch durations on hip flexion range of motion . *J Strength Cond Res* . 2010 430–436

33. Hodges PW, Richardson CA Inefficient muscular stabilization of the lumbar spine associated with low back pain A motor control evaluation of transversus abdominis . *Spine* 1996 2640–2650

34. 34. Hides J, Richardson C, Jull G Multifidus muscle recovery is not automatic after resolution of acute, first-episode low back pain Spine 1996 2763–9

35. Alfredson H, Pietila T, Jonsson P *.et al* Heavy-load eccentric calf muscle training for the treatment of chronic Achilles tendinosis *Am J Sports Med* 1998 360–366

36. Sharma P, Maffulli N Tendon Injury and Tendinopathy: Healing and Repair *The Journal of Bone and Joint Surgery American volume* 2005 187–202

37. Garg R, Adamson G, Dawson P, Shankwiler J, Pink M. A prospective randomized study comparing a forearm strap brace versus a wrist splint for the treatment of lateral epicondylitis . *Journal of Shoulder and Elbow Surgery* 2010 508–12

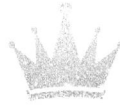

Second Edition Additional References

Alakhdar Mohmara Y, Cook J, Benítez-Martínez JC, McPeek ER, Aguilar AA, Olivas ES, Hernandez-Sanchez S. Influence of genetic factors in elbow tendon pathology: a case-control study. *Sci Rep.* 2020 Apr 16;10(1):6503.

Alfredson H, Pietilä T, Jonsson P, Lorentzon R. Heavy-load eccentric calf muscle training for the treatment of chronic Achilles tendinosis. *Am J Sports Med.* 1998 May-Jun;26(3):360–6.

Altan L., Kanat E. Conservative treatment of lateral epicondylitis: a comparison of two different orthotic devices. *Clin Rheumatol.* 2008 Aug;27(8):1015–1019.

Anderson AR, Holliday D. Mapping the associations of daily pain, sleep, and psychological distress in a U.S. sample. *J Behav Med.* 2023 Jun 29.

Balevi ISY, Karaoglan B, Batur EB, Acet N. Evaluation of short-term and residual effects of Kinesio taping in chronic lateral epicondylitis: A randomized, double-blinded, controlled trial. *J Hand Ther.* 2023 Jan-Mar;36(1):13–22.

Bargeri S, Pellicciari L, Gallo C, Rossettini G, Castellini G, Gianola S; AIFI Consortium. What is the landscape of evidence about the safety of physical agents used in physical medicine and rehabilitation? A scoping review. *BMJ Open*. 2023 Jun 23;13(6):e068134.

Barati H, Zarezadeh A, MacDermid JC, Sadeghi-Demneh E. The immediate sensorimotor effects of elbow orthoses in patients with lateral elbow tendinopathy: a prospective crossover study. *J Shoulder Elbow Surg*. 2019 Jan;28(1):e10–e17.

Basson CA, Stewart A, Mudzi W, Musenge E. Effect of Neural Mobilization on Nerve-Related Neck and Arm Pain: A Randomized Controlled Trial. *Physiother Can*. 2020 Nov 1;72(4):408–419.

Basu-Ray I. A Mechanistic Model for Yoga as a Preventive and Therapeutic Modality. *Int J Yoga*. 2021 May-Aug;14(2):152–157.

Bateman M, Littlewood C, Rawson B, Tambe AA. Surgery for tennis elbow: a systematic review. *Shoulder Elbow*. 2019 Feb;11(1):35–44.

Bazancir Z, Fırat T. A potential factor in the pathophysiology of lateral epicondylitis: The long sarcomere length of the extensor carpi radialis brevis muscle and implications for physiotherapy. *Med Hypotheses*. 2019 Sep;130:109278.

Bhabra G, Wang A, Ebert JR, Edwards P, Zheng M, Zheng MH. Lateral Elbow Tendinopathy: Development of a Pathophysiology-Based Treatment Algorithm. *Orthop J Sports Med*. 2016 Nov 1;4(11):2325967116670635.

Bisset LM, Collins NJ, Offord SS. Immediate effects of 2 types of braces on pain and grip strength in people with lateral epicondylalgia: a randomized controlled trial. *J Orthop Sports Phys Ther.* 2014 Feb;44(2):120–8.

Bonczar M, Ostrowski P, Dziedzic M, Kasprzyk M, Obuchowicz R, Zacharias T, Marchewka J, Walocha J, Koziej M. Evaluation of lateral epicondylopathy, posterior interosseous nerve compression, and plica syndrome as co-existing causes of chronic tennis elbow. *Int Orthop.* 2023 Jul;47(7):1787–1795.

Brukner P and Khan K. Elbow and arm pain. In: Bill Vicenzino B, Scott A, Bell S, Nebojsa P (eds). *Clinical sports medicine.* 4th ed. Sydney: McGraw-Hill, 2012, pp. 390–412.

Buchanan BK, Varacallo M. Tennis Elbow. [Updated 2022 Nov 7]. In: StatPearls [Internet]. Treasure Island (FL): StatPearls Publishing; 2023 Jan-. Available from: https://www.ncbi.nlm.nih.gov/books/NBK431092/

Burton I, McCormack A. Nutritional Supplements in the Clinical Management of Tendinopathy: A Scoping Review. *J Sport Rehabil.* 2023 May 5;32(5):493–504.

Bussin E, Cairns B, Gerschman T, Fredericson M, Bovard J, Scott A. Topical diclofenac vs placebo for the treatment of chronic Achilles tendinopathy: A randomized controlled clinical trial. *PLoS One.* 2021 Mar 4;16(3):e0247663.

Chaabene H, Behm DG, Negra Y, Granacher U. Acute Effects of Static Stretching on Muscle Strength and Power: An Attempt to Clarify Previous Caveats. *Front Physiol.* 2019 Nov 29;10:1468.

Cheema AS, Doyon J, Lapner P. Transcutaneous electrical nerve stimulation (TENS) and extracorporeal shockwave therapy (ESWT) in lateral epicondylitis: a systematic review and meta-analysis. *JSES Int.* 2022 Dec 10;7(2):351–356.

Chen Z, Baker NA. Effectiveness of eccentric strengthening in the treatment of lateral elbow tendinopathy: A systematic review with meta-analysis. *J Hand Ther.* 2021 Jan-Mar;34(1):18–28.

Cho YT, Hsu WY, Lin LF, Lin YN. Kinesio taping reduces elbow pain during resisted wrist extension in patients with chronic lateral epicondylitis: a randomized, double-blinded, cross over study. *BMC Musculoskelet Disord.* 2018 Jun 19;19(1):193.

Cleary MA, Sweeney LA, Kendrick ZV, Sitler MR. Dehydration and symptoms of delayed-onset muscle soreness in hyperthermic males. *J Athl Train.* 2005 Oct-Dec;40(4):288–97.

Connell D, Burke F, Coombes P, et al. Sonographic examination of lateral epicondylitis. *AJR Am J Roentgenol* 2001; 176: 777–782.

Cook JL, Rio E, Purdam CR, Docking SI. Revisiting the continuum model of tendon pathology: what is its merit in clinical practice and research? *Br J Sports Med.* 2016 Oct;50(19):1187–91.

Coombes BK, Bisset L, Brooks P, Khan A, Vicenzino B. Effect of corticosteroid injection, physiotherapy, or both on clinical outcomes in patients with unilateral lateral epicondylalgia: A randomized controlled trial. *JAMA.* 2013:461–9.

Coombes BK, Bisset L, Vicenzino B. Efficacy and safety of corticosteroid injections and other injections for management of tendinopathy: a systematic review of randomised controlled trials. *Lancet.* 2010;376:1751–1767.

Coombes BK, Wiebusch M, Heales L, Stephenson A, Vicenzino B. Isometric Exercise Above but not Below an Individual's Pain Threshold Influences Pain Perception in People With Lateral Epicondylalgia. *Clin J Pain.* 2016 Dec;32(12):1069–1075.

Cutts S, Gangoo S, Modi N, Pasapula C. Tennis elbow: A clinical review article. *J Orthop.* 2019 Aug 10;17:203–207.

Dahlhamer J, Lucas J, Zelaya C, Nahin R, Mackey S, DeBar L, Kerns R, Von Korff M, Porter L, Helmick C. Prevalence of Chronic Pain and High-Impact Chronic Pain Among Adults - United States, 2016. *MMWR Morb Mortal Wkly Rep.* 2018 Sep 14;67(36):1001–1006.

Day JM, Bush H, Nitz AJ, Uhl TL. Scapular muscle performance in individuals with lateral epicondylalgia. *J Orthop Sports Phys Ther.* 2015 May;45(5):414–24.

Descatha A, Albo F, Leclerc A, Carton M, Godeau D, Roquelaure Y, Petit A, Aublet-Cuvelier A. Lateral Epicondylitis and Physical Exposure at Work? A Review of Prospective Studies and Meta-Analysis. *Arthritis Care Res (Hoboken).* 2016 Nov;68(11):1681–1687.

Dingemanse R, Randsdorp M, Koes BW, Huisstede BM Evidence for the effectiveness of electrophysical modalities for treatment of medial and lateral epicondylitis: a systematic review. *Br J Sports Med.* 2014 957–65.

Dragan S, Șerban MC, Damian G, Buleu F, Valcovici M, Christodorescu R. Dietary Patterns and Interventions to Alleviate Chronic Pain. *Nutrients.* 2020 Aug 19;12(9):2510.

El-Leithy, S.A., Adly, N.N. & Galal, S. Role of vitamin D in lateral epicondylitis among Egyptians. *Egypt Rheumatol Rehabil* 50, 61 (2023).

Ellis R, Carta G, Andrade RJ, Coppieters MW. Neurodynamics: is tension contentious? *J Man Manip Ther.* 2022 Feb;30(1):3–12.

Eraslan L, Yuce D, Erbilici A, Baltaci G. Does Kinesiotaping improve pain and functionality in patients with newly diagnosed lateral epicondylitis? *Knee Surg Sports Traumatol Arthrosc.* 2018 Mar;26(3):938–945.

Fahlström M, Jonsson P, Lorentzon R, Alfredson H. Chronic Achilles tendon pain treated with eccentric calf-muscle training. *Knee Surg Sports Traumatol Arthrosc.* 2003 Sep;11(5):327–33.

George CE, Heales LJ, Stanton R, et al. Sticking to the facts: a systematic review of the effects of therapeutic tape in lateral epicondylalgia. *Phys Ther Sport* 2019; 40: 117–127.

Giray E, Karali-Bingul D, Akyuz G. The Effectiveness of Kinesiotaping, Sham Taping or Exercises Only in Lateral Epicondylitis Treatment: A Randomized Controlled Study. *PM R.* 2019 Jul;11(7):681–693.

Green S., Buchbinder R., Barnsley L., Hall S., White M., Smidt N., Assendelft W. Non-steroidal anti-inflammatory drugs (NSAIDs) for treating lateral elbow pain in adults. *Cochrane Database Syst Rev.* 2002 (2):CD003686.

Hall A, Copsey B, Richmond H, Thompson J, Ferreira M, Latimer J, Maher CG. Effectiveness of Tai Chi for Chronic Musculoskeletal Pain Conditions: Updated Systematic Review and Meta-Analysis. *Phys Ther.* 2017 Feb 1;97(2):227–238.

Hay E.M., Paterson S., Lewish M. Croft P Pragmatic randomised controlled trial of local corticosteroid injection and naproxen for treatment of lateral epicondylitis of elbow in primary care. *BMJ.* 1999;319:964–968.

Heales LJ, Bergin MJG, Vicenzino B, Hodges PW. Forearm Muscle Activity in Lateral Epicondylalgia: A Systematic Review with Quantitative Analysis. *Sports Med.* 2016 Dec;46(12):1833–1845.

Heales LJ, Bout N, Dines B, Parker T, Reddiex K, Kean CO, Obst SJ. An Investigation of Maximal Strength of the Upper Limb Bilaterally in Individuals With Lateral Elbow Tendinopathy: A Systematic Review With Meta-Analysis. *Phys Ther.* 2021 Dec 1;101(12):pzab230.

Heales LJ, Lim EC, Hodges PW, Vicenzino B. Sensory and motor deficits exist on the non-injured side of patients with unilateral tendon pain and disability--implications for central nervous system involvement: a systematic review with meta-analysis. *Br J Sports Med.* 2014 Oct;48(19):1400–6.

Heales LJ, McClintock SR, Maynard S, Lems CJ, Rose JA, Hill C, Kean CO, Obst S. Evaluating the immediate effect of forearm and wrist orthoses on pain and function in individuals with lateral elbow tendinopathy: A systematic review. *Musculoskelet Sci Pract.* 2020 Jun;47:102147.

Herquelot E, Guéguen A, Roquelaure Y, Bodin J, Sérazin C, Ha C, Leclerc A, Goldberg M, Zins M, Descatha A. Work-related risk factors for incidence of lateral epicondylitis in a large working population. *Scand J Work Environ Health.* 2013 Nov;39(6):578–88.

Hijlkema A, Roozenboom C, Mensink M, Zwerver J. The impact of nutrition on tendon health and tendinopathy: a systematic review. *J Int Soc Sports Nutr.* 2022 Aug 3;19(1):474–504.

Hill CE, Heales LJ, Stanton R, Kean CO. Effects of multidirectional elastic tape on pain and function in individuals with lateral elbow tendinopathy: A randomised crossover trial. *Clinical Rehabilitation.* 2023;37(8):1041–1051.

Hoogvliet P, Randsdorp MS, Dingemanse R, Koes BW, Huisstede BM. Does effectiveness of exercise therapy and mobilisation techniques offer guidance for the treatment of lateral and medial epicondylitis? A systematic review. *Br J Sports Med.* 2013 Nov;47(17):1112–9.

Jalovaara P., Lindholm R.V. Decompression of the posterior interosseous nerve for tennis elbo. *Arch Orthop Trauma Surg.* July 1989;108(4):243–245.

Janela D, Costa F, Molinos M, Moulder RG, Lains J, Bento V, Scheer JK, Yanamadala V, Cohen SP, Correia FD. Digital Rehabilitation for Elbow Pain Musculoskeletal Conditions: A Prospective Longitudinal Cohort Study. *Int J Environ Res Public Health.* 2022 Jul 27;19(15):9198.

Järvinen TA. Neovascularisation in tendinopathy: from eradication to stabilisation? *Br J Sports Med.* 2020 Jan;54(1):1–2.

Jerger S, Centner C, Lauber B, et al. Effects of specific collagen peptide supplementation combined with resistance training on Achilles tendon properties. *Scand J Med Sci Sports.* 2022; 32: 1131–1141.

Jespersen A, Amris K, Graven-Nielsen T, Arendt-Nielsen L, Bartels EM, Torp-Pedersen S, Bliddal H, Danneskiold-Samsoe B. Assessment of pressure-pain thresholds and central sensitization of pain in lateral epicondylalgia. *Pain Med.* 2013;14:297–304.

Johns N, Shridhar V. Lateral epicondylitis: Current concepts. *Aust J Gen Pract.* 2020 Nov;49(11):707–709.

Juul-Kristensen B, Lund H, Hansen K, Christensen H, Danneskiold-Samsøe B, Bliddal H. Poorer elbow proprioception in patients with lateral epicondylitis than in healthy controls: a cross-sectional study. *J Shoulder Elbow Surg.* 2008 Jan-Feb;17(1 Suppl):72S–81S.

Karabinov V, Georgiev GP. Lateral epicondylitis: New trends and challenges in treatment. *World J Orthop.* 2022 Apr 18;13(4):354–364.

Karjalainen TV, Silagy M, O'Bryan E, Johnston RV, Cyril S, Buchbinder R. Autologous blood and platelet-rich plasma injection therapy for lateral elbow pain. *Cochrane Database Syst Rev.* 2021 Sep 30;9(9):CD010951.

Keijsers R, de Vos RJ, Kuijer PPF, van den Bekerom MP, van der Woude HJ, Eygendaal D. Tennis elbow. *Shoulder Elbow.* 2019 Oct;11(5):384–392.

Kim YJ, Wood SM, Yoon AP, Howard JC, Yang LY, Chung KC. Efficacy of Nonoperative Treatments for Lateral Epicondylitis: A Systematic Review and Meta-Analysis. *Plast Reconstr Surg.* 2021 Jan 1;147(1):112–125.

Knobloch K. Eccentric training in Achilles tendinopathy: is it harmful to tendon microcirculation? *Br J Sports Med.* 2007 Jun;41(6).

Kong LJ, Lauche R, Klose P, Bu JH, Yang XC, Guo CQ, Dobos G, Cheng YW. Tai Chi for Chronic Pain Conditions: A Systematic Review and Meta-analysis of Randomized Controlled Trials. *Sci Rep.* 2016 Apr 29;6:25325.

Kroslak M, Pirapakaran K, Murrell GAC. Counterforce bracing of lateral epicondylitis: a prospective, randomized, double-blinded, placebo-controlled clinical trial. *J Shoulder Elbow Surg.* 2019 Feb;28(2):288–95.

Lai WC, Erickson BJ, Mlynarek RA, Wang D. Chronic lateral epicondylitis: challenges and solutions. *Open Access J Sports Med.* 2018 Oct 30;9:243–251.

Le Huec, Schaeverbeke T., Chauveaux D., Rivel J., Dehias J., Le Rebekker A.L. Epicondylitis after treatment with fluoroquinolone Antibiotics. *J Bone Joint Surg Br Vol.* March 1995;77-B(2):293–295.

Li IC, Lee LY, Tzeng TT, Chen WP, Chen YP, Shiao YJ, Chen CC. Neurohealth Properties of *Hericium erinaceus* Mycelia Enriched with Erinacines. *Behav Neurol.* 2018 May 21;2018:5802634.

Li Q. Effect of forest bathing trips on human immune function. *Environ Health Prev Med.* 2010 Jan;15(1):9–17.

Li ZJ, Yang QQ, Zhou YL. Basic Research on Tendon Repair: Strategies, Evaluation, and Development. *Front Med* (Lausanne). 2021 Jul 28;8:664909.

Linnanmäki L, Kanto K, Karjalainen T, Leppänen OV, Lehtinen J. Platelet-rich Plasma or Autologous Blood Do Not Reduce Pain or Improve Function in Patients with Lateral Epicondylitis: A Randomized Controlled Trial. *Clin Orthop Relat Res.* 2020 Aug;478(8):1892–1900.

Mafi N, Lorentzon R, Alfredson H. Superior short-term results with eccentric calf muscle training compared to concentric training in a randomized prospective multicenter study on patients with chronic Achilles tendinosis. *Knee Surg Sports Traumatol Arthrosc.* 2001;9(1):42–7.

Manias P., Stasinopolous D. A controlled clinical pilot trial to study the effectiveness of ice as a supplement to the exercise programme for the management of lateral elbow tedinopathy. *Br J Sports Med.* 2006 Jan;40(1):81–85.

McCall T. New York: Bantam Dell a division of Random House Inc; 2007. *Yoga as Medicine.*

McCallum SD, Paoloni JA, Murrell GA. Five-year prospective comparison study of topical glyceryl trinitrate treatment of chronic lateral epicondylosis at the elbow. *Br J Sports Med.* 2011 Apr;45(5):416–20.

McCartney D, Benson MJ, Desbrow B, Irwin C, Suraev A, McGregor IS. Cannabidiol and Sports Performance: a Narrative Review of Relevant Evidence and Recommendations for Future Research. *Sports Med Open.* 2020 Jul 6;6(1):27.

Nirschl RP. The epidemiology and health care burden of tennis elbow: a population-based study. *Ann Transl Med.* 2015 Jun;3(10):133.

Noriega-González DC, Drobnic F, Caballero-García A, Roche E, Perez-Valdecantos D, Córdova A. Effect of Vitamin C on Tendinopathy Recovery: A Scoping Review. *Nutrients.* 2022 Jun 27;14(13):2663.

Nuñez de Arenas-Arroyo S, Martínez-Vizcaíno V, Cavero-Redondo I, Álvarez-Bueno C, Reina-Gutierrez S, Torres-Costoso A. The Effect of Neurodynamic Techniques on the Dispersion of Intraneural Edema: A Systematic Review with Meta-Analysis. *Int J Environ Res Public Health.* 2022 Nov 4;19(21):14472.

O'Dowd A. Update on the Use of Platelet-Rich Plasma Injections in the Management of Musculoskeletal Injuries: A Systematic Review of Studies From 2014 to 2021. *Orthop J Sports Med.* 2022 Dec 9;10(12):23259671221140888.

Ohberg L, Lorentzon R, Alfredson H. Eccentric training in patients with chronic Achilles tendinosis: normalised tendon structure and decreased thickness at follow up. *Br J Sports Med.* 2004;38:8–11.

Ortega-Castillo M, Cuesta-Vargas A, Luque-Teba A, Trinidad-Fernández M. The role of progressive, therapeutic exercise in the management of upper limb tendinopathies: A systematic review and meta-analysis. *Musculoskelet Sci Pract.* 2022 Dec;62:102645.

Ortega-Castillo M, Medina-Porqueres I. Effectiveness of the eccentric exercise therapy in physically active adults with symptomatic shoulder impingement or lateral epicondylar tendinopathy: A systematic review. *J Sci Med Sport.* 2016 Jun;19(6):438–53.

Öte Karaca Ş, Demirsoy N, Günendi Z. Effects of aerobic exercise on pain sensitivity, heart rate recovery, and health-related quality of life in patients with chronic musculoskeletal pain. *Int J Rehabil Res.* 2017 Jun;40(2):164–170.

Palmer KL, Shivgulam ME, Champod AS, Wilson BC, O'Brien MW, Bray NW. Exercise training augments brain function and reduces pain perception in adults with chronic pain: A systematic review of intervention studies. *Neurobiol Pain.* 2023 Apr 20;13:100129.

Park HB, Gwark JY, Im JH, Na JB. Factors Associated With Lateral Epicondylitis of the Elbow. *Orthop J Sports Med.* 2021 May 13;9(5):23259671211007734.

Pattanittum P, Turner T, Green S, Buchbinder R. Non-steroidal anti-inflammatory drugs (NSAIDs) for treating lateral elbow pain in adults. *Cochrane Database Syst Rev.* 2013 May 31;2013(5):CD003686.

Peterson M, Butler S, Eriksson M, Svärdsudd K. A randomized controlled trial of eccentric vs. concentric graded exercise in chronic tennis elbow (lateral elbow tendinopathy). *Clin Rehabil.* 2014 Sep;28(9):862–72.

Previtali D, Mameli A, Zaffagnini S, Marchettini P, Candrian C, Filardo G. Tendinopathies and Pain Sensitisation: A Meta-Analysis with Meta-Regression. *Biomedicines.* 2022 Jul 20;10(7):1749.

Radecka A, Lubkowska A. Direct Effect of Local Cryotherapy on Muscle Stimulation, Pain and Strength in Male Office Workers with Lateral Epicondylitis, Non-Randomized Clinical Trial Study. *Healthcare (Basel).* 2022 May 10;10(5):879.

Raffaeli W, Tenti M, Corraro A, Malafoglia V, Ilari S, Balzani E, Bonci A. Chronic Pain: What Does It Mean? A Review on the Use of the Term Chronic Pain in Clinical Practice. *J Pain Res.* 2021 Mar 29;14:827–835.

Reuter S. Physiotherapeutische Möglichkeiten bei lateraler Epikondylopathie [Physiotherapeutic therapy modalities for lateral epicondyopathy]. *Orthopadie (Heidelb).* 2023 May;52(5):359–364.

Rio E, Kidgell D, Moseley GL, Gaida J, Docking S, Purdam C, Cook J. Tendon neuroplastic training: changing the way we think about tendon rehabilitation: a narrative review. *Br J Sports Med.* 2016 Feb;50(4):209–15.

Sabaratnam V, Kah-Hui W, Naidu M, Rosie David P. Neuronal health - can culinary and medicinal mushrooms help? *J Tradit Complement Med.* 2013 Jan;3(1):62–8.

Savnik A., Jensen B., Norregaard J., Egund N., Danneskiold-Samsoe B., Bliddal H. Magnetic resonance imaging in the evaluation of treatment response of lateral epicondylitis of the elbow. *Eur Radiol.* 2004 Jun;14(6):964–969.

Schiffke-Juhász, B. & Knobloch, Karsten & Vogt, Peter & Hoy, L.. Proprioceptive elbow training reduces pain and improves function in painful lateral epicondylitis—a prospective trial. *Journal of Orthopaedic Surgery and Research.* 2021 Jul;16(10):1186.

Sethi K, Noohu MM. Scapular muscles strengthening on pain, functional outcome and muscle activity in chronic lateral epicondylalgia. *J Orthop Sci.* 2018 Sep;23(5):777–782.

Shahabi S, Bagheri Lankarani K, Heydari ST, et al. The effects of counterforce brace on pain in subjects with lateral elbow tendinopathy: A systematic review and meta-analysis of randomized controlled trials. *Prosthetics and Orthotics International.* 2020;44(5):341–354.

Simental-Mendía M, Vilchez-Cavazos F, Álvarez-Villalobos N, Blázquez-Saldaña J, Peña-Martínez V, Villarreal-Villarreal G, Acosta-Olivo C. Clinical efficacy of platelet-rich plasma in the treatment of lateral epicondylitis: a systematic review and meta-analysis of randomized placebo-controlled clinical trials. *Clin Rheumatol.* 2020 Aug;39(8):2255–2265.

Speers CJ, Bhogal GS, Collins R. Lateral elbow tendinosis: a review of diagnosis and management in general practice. *Br J Gen Pract.* 2018 Nov;68(676):548–549.

Stasinopoulos D. Lateral elbow tendinopathy: Evidence of physiotherapy management. *World J Orthop.* 2016 Aug 18;7(8):463–6.

Stasinopoulos D. The role of proprioception in the management of lateral elbow tendinopathy. *J Hand Ther.* 2019 Jan-Mar;32(1):e2-e3.

Stasinopoulos D. Isometric Exercise for the Management of Lateral Elbow Tendinopathy. *J Clin Med.* 2022 Dec 22;12(1):94.

Takahashi I, Matsuzaki T, Kuroki H, Hoso M. Disuse Atrophy of Articular Cartilage Induced by Unloading Condition Accelerates Histological Progression of Osteoarthritis in a Post-traumatic Rat Model. *Cartilage.* 2021 Dec;13(2_suppl):1522S–1529S.

Tan L, Cicuttini FM, Fairley J, Romero L, Estee M, Hussain SM, Urquhart DM. Does aerobic exercise effect pain sensitisation in individuals with musculoskeletal pain? A systematic review. *BMC Musculoskelet Disord.* 2022 Feb 3;23(1):113.

Treede RD, Rief W, Barke A, Aziz Q, Bennett MI, Benoliel R, Cohen M, Evers S, Finnerup NB, First MB, Giamberardino MA, Kaasa S, Kosek E, Lavand'homme P, Nicholas M, Perrot S, Scholz J, Schug S, Smith BH, Svensson P, Vlaeyen JWS, Wang SJ. A classification of chronic pain for ICD-11. *Pain.* 2015 Jun;156(6):1003–1007.

Turnagöl IIH, Koşar ŞN, Güzel Y, Aktitiz S, Atakan MM. Nutritional Considerations for Injury Prevention and Recovery in Combat Sports. *Nutrients.* 2021 Dec 23;14(1):53.

Ucurum SG, Karabay D, Ozturk BB, Kaya DO. Comparison of scapular position and upper extremity muscle strength in patients with and without lateral epicondylalgia: a case-control study. *J Shoulder Elbow Surg.* 2019 Jun;28(6):1111–1119.

Unverferth LJ, Olix ML. The Effect of Local Steroid Injections on Tendon. *J Sports Med.* 1973;1:31–37.

Vicenzino B. Lateral epicondylalgia: a musculoskeletal physiotherapy perspective. *Man Ther.* 2003 May;8(2):66–79.

Wen Y, Yan Q, Pan Y, Gu X, Liu Y. Medical empirical research on forest bathing (Shinrin-yoku): a systematic review. *Environ Health Prev Med.* 2019 Dec 1;24(1):70.

Welsh P. Tendon neuroplastic training for lateral elbow tendinopathy: 2 case reports. *J Can Chiropr Assoc.* 2018 Aug;62(2):98–104.

Weston-Green K, Clunas H, Jimenez Naranjo C. A Review of the Potential Use of Pinene and Linalool as Terpene-Based Medicines for Brain Health: Discovering Novel Therapeutics in the Flavours and Fragrances of Cannabis. *Front Psychiatry*. 2021 Aug 26;12:583211.

Woodyard C. Exploring the therapeutic effects of yoga and its ability to increase quality of life. *Int J Yoga*. 2011 Jul;4(2):49–54.

Xu J, Chen M, Xue X, Zhou W, Luo X. Global Research Trends and Hotspots in Lateral Epicondylitis During the Past 30 Years: A Bibliometric and Visualization Study. *Med Sci Monit*. 2023 May 28;29:e939309.

Yalcin A, Kayaalp ME. Comparison of Hyaluronate & Steroid Injection in the Treatment of Chronic Lateral Epicondylitis and Evaluation of Treatment Efficacy With MRI: A Single-Blind, Prospective, Randomized Controlled Clinical Study. *Cureus*. 2022 Sep 10;14(9):e29011.

Yang S, Chang MC. Chronic Pain: Structural and Functional Changes in Brain Structures and Associated Negative Affective States. *Int J Mol Sci*. 2019 Jun 26;20(13):3130.

Yoon SY, Kim YW, Shin IS, Kang S, Moon HI, Lee SC. The Beneficial Effects of Eccentric Exercise in the Management of Lateral Elbow Tendinopathy: A Systematic Review and Meta-Analysis. *J Clin Med*. 2021 Sep 1;10(17):3968.

Yoon SY, Kim YW, Shin IS, Moon HI, Lee SC. Does the Type of Extracorporeal Shock Therapy Influence Treatment Effectiveness in Lateral Epicondylitis? A Systematic Review and Meta-analysis. *Clin Orthop Relat Res*. 2020 Oct;478(10):2324–2339.

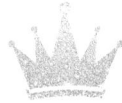

Acknowledgments

This book would not be in your hands but for the following people:

- My family for bearing with me whilst I wrote this book - again! I know it was tough at times, boys, but we made it through - again!

- Buddy Gibbons, the inspiration for finding the solution to tennis elbow and going along with my different ideas until we got it right! I love that we are still in each other's lives.

- Dr Annette Billings for entrusting me with her wonderful clients and her deep friendship. It still means more to me than you know.

- Leesa Ellis, my book mentor, for holding my hand through the process of writing my first book, my second book and the second edition of my first book! I could not have done any of this without your guidance!

- John Takemura, for taking a chance on a crazy English physio and putting her in an office with Jackie Chipot!

- Beth Moser Chang for the amazing photos, thank you friend. Your work astounds me every time.

- Sam Griffiths for the wonderful illustration and my Tennis Elbow Queen logo. You truly are Miss Chief Creative.

- The pre-readers who gave me frank and valuable advice on how best to present this information.

- The participants of my program who tested new elements that research brought forth.

- And of course, the readers of the first edition who gave me the feedback and incentive to improve this book. Thank you!

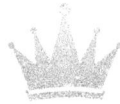

About the Author

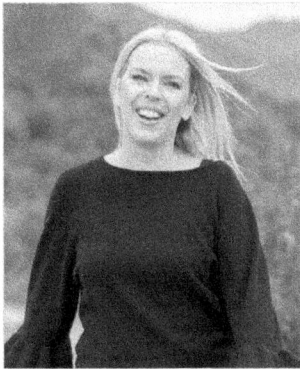

Emma Green, the Tennis Elbow Queen, is a 30-year physical therapist based in Los Angeles. With a wealth of experience in the field, she is a former professional sports PT, best-selling author of *Tennis Elbow Relief* and *Get Out Of Pain Fast!* and is the creator of the Comprehensive Elbow Pain Relief Program, which has transformed the lives of thousands of tennis elbow sufferers around the world.

Emma graduated from Manchester University, England as a Physical Therapist and added a Master's degree in Sports Injury and Therapy. Prior to TennisElbowQueen.com, Emma began her career in the UK as a professional sports PT, the highlight of which was working at the London 2012 Olympic Games. Currently, her virtual practice focuses on the treatment of individuals with tennis elbow.

Emma has presented at numerous conferences around the globe and is a Certified Instructor for Empowered Relief® through Stanford University and a Certified High-Performance Coach through the High Performance Institute. Emma's extensive knowledge and dedication to her field make her a trusted source of information on tennis elbow.

Emma enjoys running (has just completed her second marathon), traveling extensively and spending time with her family.

Find her at:
https://www.TennisElbowQueen.com

Facebook:
https://www.facebook.com/TennisElbowQueenPT

Instagram:
https://www.instagram.com/tenniselbowqueen/

YouTube:
https://www.youtube.com/c/
EmmaGreenTennisElbowQueen

www.ingramcontent.com/pod-product-compliance
Lightning Source LLC
Chambersburg PA
CBHW051244020426
42333CB00025B/3046